I have had the opportunity to lecture around the world for the past twenty-five years and have so enjoyed meeting many thousands of orthodontists, often visiting their office while treating their patients. On many occasions, I have had the pleasure of visiting the Mesa office and am so impressed with how Dr. Frost and his outstanding staff exhibit such professionalism and a strong desire to create the most beautiful smiles in the world in a remarkably short period of time. It is obvious that their focus is on producing the highest quality of patient care utilizing the most advanced technologies that feature the application of very healthy biologic forces. I can honestly say that I have never met a more focused and talented clinician in my many years in this wonderful profession.

Dr. Frost's goals are far more than just achieving straight teeth. His incredible talent allows him to create incredible smiles with facial beauty and balance for the patient's lifetime. The Phoenix area is very fortunate to have a clinician of Dr. Frost's caliber. I can only give him the very highest recommendation because he is truly an extraordinarily talented clinician with great passion, and he cares for each patient he has the pleasure of giving an amazing, world-class smile.

DR. DWIGHT DAMON
INVENTOR OF THE DAMON SYSTEM

T0273536

When it comes to creating beautiful smiles, even those of us who lecture beside Dr. Frost are amazed at the artistry with which he practices his craft. A master at combining the art and science of orthodontics, the smiles he creates are recognizable worldwide. For the patients lucky enough to visit his practice, the results are obvious. What many of these patients don't know is that the entire orthodontic profession benefits from Dr. Frost's expertise through his insightful teaching. As an internationally renowned orthodontic educator, Dr. Frost has lectured on the largest of world stages, educating thousands of orthodontists on his masterful style of artistic orthodontic treatment. Countless patients around the world benefit from his selfless sharing of his years of experience and insight. I'm proud to call Dr. Frost my friend and mentor, and I know my orthodontic expertise has been enhanced by learning from him over the past decade!

DR. JEFF KOZLOWSKI

There are those in a given field who are exceptional and admired. Then there are those that are so revered that they elevate the field to new heights. Dr. Stuart Frost is the latter. I'm fortunate to have rubbed shoulders with most of the clinical giants of orthodontics, and hands down, Dr. Frost is at the top of those giants.

JOHN. W. GRAHAM, DDS, MD
SALT LAKE CITY, UTAH

"I am fortunate to have been in orthodontics since the turn of the millennium. Over my career, I have attended meetings, watched speakers, and met clinicians from all over the world. However, among the doctors I have met, watched, or learned from, I have the honor of calling a select, elite few my mentors. Those doctors I respect for their integrity and clinical skill above all others. I can honestly say, I have never met a finer orthodontist and innovator than Dr. Stuart Frost. He is truly one of the most gifted individuals in our profession and he has my highest recommendation."

DR. JAMIE REYNOLDS

Dr. Frost has been my close friend and mentor for more than fifteen years. It was his passion, dedication, selflessness, and excellence in treatment that inspired me to become an orthodontist. I have never met another individual with the capacity to freely give so much of himself for the betterment of others. Dr. Frost is the kind of orthodontist that continues to inspire, in and out of the mouth. His passion for both the field of orthodontics, and his artistry as a clinician, are unmatched by any doctor I have met. As a resident, he is everything I hope to become as an orthodontist. Dr. Frost has a special ability that is well-known by all in the community to serve and uplift. His "smile brand" is something I seek after for each of my patients, and something that he has mastered. He truly has a zest for life that is contagious to all he meets. Dr. Frost is the kind of mentor that you never forget, and one you always hope to make proud!

DR. TREVOR NICHOLS

THE artist ORTHODONTIST

THE
artist
ORTHODONTIST

Creating an artistic smile
is more than just straightening teeth!

STUART FROST, DDS

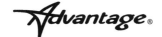

Published by Advantage, Charleston, South Carolina.
Member of Advantage Media Group.

ADVANTAGE is a registered trademark, and the Advantage colophon is a trademark of Advantage Media Group, Inc.

Printed in the United States of America.

10 9 8 7 6 5 4 3 2 1

ISBN: 978-1-59932-949-9
LCCN: 2018948457

Book design by Carly Blake.

This publication is designed to provide accurate and authoritative information in regard to the subject matter covered. It is sold with the understanding that the publisher is not engaged in rendering legal, accounting, or other professional services. If legal advice or other expert assistance is required, the services of a competent professional person should be sought.

Advantage Media Group is proud to be a part of the Tree Neutral® program. Tree Neutral offsets the number of trees consumed in the production and printing of this book by taking proactive steps such as planting trees in direct proportion to the number of trees used to print books. To learn more about Tree Neutral, please visit **www.treeneutral.com**.

Advantage Media Group is a publisher of business, self-improvement, and professional development books and online learning. We help entrepreneurs, business leaders, and professionals share their Stories, Passion, and Knowledge to help others Learn & Grow. Do you have a manuscript or book idea that you would like us to consider for publishing? Please visit **advantagefamily.com** or call **1.866.775.1696**.

This book is dedicated to my mom and dad, who made me share every-thing in life. What a gift! To my wife, Christina, who breathed life back into my soul. To my twin brother, Steve, with whom I share a strong competitive spirit that drives us both to excel in our professions. Everyone should have a twin! To my friend-brother-colleague, Dr. James Russell Glauser, you are still larger than life, and terribly missed! To my high school football coach, Jessie Parker, who taught me mental toughness and that I could do anything for five seconds.

Table of Contents

Preface

Art was not my favorite subject in school. In fact, I am not good at drawing or painting and my handwriting is a little like chicken scratch. So you can imagine my surprise when someone referred to me as an *artist*.

The day my family had a family photo taken changed my career forever. I have always had a passion for smiles and straight teeth, but the day I met the photographer Allison Tyler Jones changed my perception of myself as an orthodontist. She made one simple comment: "I know who you are. You are known as the artist orthodontist."

I didn't know what to say, because I had never considered myself an artist. I asked her how she knew that.

She simply replied, "I have been taking photographs of all your patients and many of the other orthodontists' patients in the community and your smiles are works of art."

My self-perception changed that day. I am an artist orthodontist! A beautiful smile is a work of art. Though I had never considered myself an artist, I realized, that day, that I too can see a beautiful orthodontic smile before a bracket is ever placed in the mouth and on a tooth, just as an artist can see the end result before the brush strokes the canvas. I love the creative process and have a passion for designing and molding beautiful smiles.

I call each smile I create a Frostsmile, as if it were the title of a work of art.

The Artist Orthodontist

Don't cry because it's over;
smile because it happened.
~ DR. SEUSS

love orthodontics and creating beautiful smiles. That passion has been ingrained in me from when I was a teenager and my dentist-father experimented on my smile with clear braces on my front teeth. The day he put those braces on my teeth, I thought I was the coolest kid in town. I was smitten! The day he took my braces off was even more incredible. It transformed me. I loved my new smile. It was at that defining moment that I realized I didn't want to just be a dentist; I wanted to be an orthodontist! I wanted to transform lives.

Fast forward to a beautiful, sunny, fall afternoon in Arizona. It's four in the afternoon on a Monday and I just removed the braces from one of my most challenging but rewarding cases. I reflected on the day Mindy showed up in my consultation room. She had braces as a teenager and her treatment had consisted of having eight permanent teeth extracted and wearing braces for well over two years. Due to new technology in braces, most of my current patients will never have to experience what Mindy went through as a teenager, with all those extractions and that length of treatment.

Almost thirty years later, Mindy heard about new technology that widens and broadens smiles with fewer extractions and requires less treatment time. She contacted me to discuss whether that technology might be the answer to "getting her smile back." People often make this request because of facial changes that occur due to the natural effects of aging, which may be compounded by changes to the structure of their face caused by earlier treatments or tooth loss.

I have always had the latest and greatest technologies in my practice. Today, those include an i-CAT 3-D x-ray, a professional photography studio, 3-D scanners, 3-D printers, and the latest technology in braces and wires. Using these technologies to evaluate Mindy's facial features, I noticed that her lip and midface bore the aftermath of many extractions. Her profile was flat and her upper lip was sunken in and didn't have much lip support. That type of facial feature would only worsen as she aged, and she was concerned about how that would affect her smile over time. After a comprehensive exam and review of her records, I presented Mindy with a treatment plan that would widen her smile and enhance her facial features—and would give her back her smile.

After I removed her braces and smoothed, contoured, and polished her teeth, I handed her a mirror to show her the final results.

She took the mirror, raised it up, and stared into it with no expression for what seemed like an eternity. Then the tears started to flow. I wasn't sure what the tears meant until she raised her hand, touched her face, and said, "I have my smile back." She was so happy, and I realized those were happy tears.

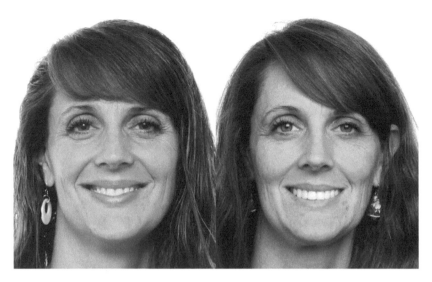

BEFORE   AFTER

After her appointment, I walked back to my private office. My thoughts turned to my childhood experience, and especially to my father, the man who had inspired me.

I reminded myself, again, that what had happened with Mindy is why I chose this amazing profession. Giving patients their smile back, and creating a spectacular, artistic smile and facial features are what drive me on a daily basis. It is exactly the life I imagined when my father transformed my smile when I was a teenager many years ago. This is what I do.

To this day, each time I remove a set of braces, I am reminded of how much I love this profession and how much I love my father for setting me on this path.

A beautiful smile is a work of art!

A SIMPLER TIME

I grew up in the 1970s, an era when a milkman delivered milk to our doorstep, the television had rabbit-ears antennae that were adjusted to tune the channel, and the brother-and-sister team of Donnie and Marie Osmond had a hit TV show. Life was simple.

My dad was a dentist and my mother was a schoolteacher. My mother had an amazing smile that caused others to instantly smile back—I can still see her smile in my mind today. When I entered the world, my family already included three children under age six. Thirty-eight weeks into her pregnancy with me, and concerned that she was larger than with past pregnancies, my mom got some surprise news from her doctor: she was having *twins*. Imagine raising five kids under age six. She delivered two, six-pound, identical twin boys. I am four minutes older than my twin brother, Steve. When delivered, we looked so alike that the nurses had to mark my foot to be able to tell us apart.

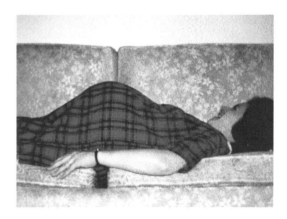

Have you ever wanted to be a twin or wondered what it would be like to have someone who looks, talks, and acts as you do and is also your best friend? Let me share with you what it's like.

Steve and I did everything together when we were growing up. When people hear that I am an identical twin, one of the first questions they ask is whether we played tricks on people, since it was so hard to tell us apart. In fact, during our senior year of high school, we decided to switch classes and see if anyone could tell. I will never forget that day because I went to Steve's sex-education class and he went to my English class. Even though he had to give a spontaneous oral report (for which he got an A), the teacher had no idea it wasn't me. Our friends knew we had switched classes, but the teachers never found out about it.

Our senior year, our dad bought us a '77 Pontiac Trans Am, *Smokey and the Bandit*-style, that bore the license plate CNDBL, (which stands for "seein' double ").

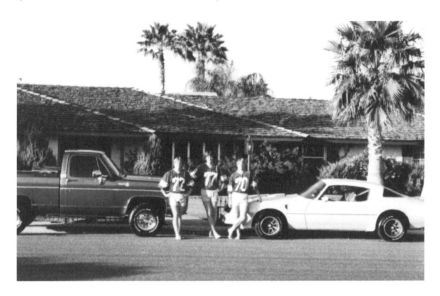

As many twins do, we bonded on most things (we gave our parents the run for their money), but we also shared a strong competitive spirit. That intense and ongoing comparison we shared was a driving force that pushed each of us to excel in anything we set out to accomplish.

Even after high school, we continued to follow the same path in life: we went to the same undergrad and dental school at the University of the Pacific in San Francisco. It was only after dental school that we chose different paths. As kids, my brother and I hung around our father's general dentistry office, watching him work and getting into mischief in his dental lab, where we would melt wax and drill plastic teeth. It is a miracle we didn't burn the office down.

We both wanted to be like our father. Back then, my brother was determined to work with our father while I wanted to specialize in orthodontics. But while we were in dental school together, my brother proved to be almost a savant at root canals, which inspired him to immediately enter a specialty program in endodontics. I, on the other hand, went to work in our father's practice for a few years following dental school before entering my orthodontic residency as I had originally intended. I will always cherish my five years, working side by side with such an amazing dentist and father.

A CALLING TO IMPROVE ORTHODONTICS ON A GRAND SCALE

The person who follows the crowd will usually go no further than the crowd. The person who walks alone is likely to find himself in places no one has ever seen before.
~ ALBERT EINSTEIN

I come from a family of dentists. In addition to my father and my brother, my brothers-in-law include a general dentist, an endodontist, an oral surgeon, and a nephew who is a pediatric dentist. As I write this book, my twin brother and I each have sons who are applying to dental school. It's a family tradition!

More than a beloved, long-time dentist, my father was a pioneer in implant dentistry. He was continually learning all he could in order to better himself for his patients. He did implants back in the late 1960s and early 1970s, when implants were still in the experimental stage.

I was ultimately inspired to be the best at orthodontics after watching him on his journey to improve implant dentistry and bless patients' lives by restoring occlusions (how teeth come into contact) and teeth lost by a multitude of problems.

While practicing dentistry with him in the early 1990s, I began to notice some issues with patients who had already undergone orthodontic treatment. A large number of patients had undergone *painful tooth extractions*, other *invasive procedures*, and *long treatment times* that had lasted in excess of four or more years. These patients were showing signs of *bone loss, root reabsorption, and receding gums.* Later in my understanding of orthodontics, I realized these problems were caused by high-force orthodontics using older braces technology. Many adults I see today were treated with those old-technology braces, and they often comment that during their previous treatment, their teeth hurt for several days after an adjustment. Many even describe the experience as so painful that they don't want their children to go through what they did.

I felt the profession needed to be further along than it was, and I was hoping that in going back to school for orthodontics, I might find that there were better ways of treating patients. In addition to the orthodontic residency, I chose to do a one-year fellowship in treating disorders of the temporomandibular joint (TMJ). That gave me a background on how the jaw functions, how it relates to teeth, and how braces might help people who suffer with jaw popping, joint noises, jaw pain, and sometimes, jaws that get stuck open or closed.

During my first year of orthodontic residency, I met a true pioneer in orthodontics, someone whose techniques were unlike any I had ever known before. I was so thirsty for information and had such high hopes for finding innovation and technology changes in orthodontics that when the opportunity arose to hear a presentation by Dr. Dwight Damon, the pioneer of passive, self-ligation brackets, I sat in the front row. It had been one hundred years since an innovation had changed the way orthodontics moved teeth, and I couldn't wait to see what his innovation was all about. His new bracket system meant *fewer extractions, less root reabsorption, fewer problems with the gums, and shorter treatment times.* His technology, the Damon System, struck a chord with me immediately because those were all the problems I was witnessing in my general dentistry practice. Although I didn't know it at the time, seeing the results of his new system demonstrated on various patients wasn't just about lining up the front teeth and giving the patient a good bite. He had the most beautiful orthodontic cases that I'd ever seen. He must have shown fifty cases in the presentation. In every case, the gum tissue and teeth were flawless—every one of those smiles and faces was beautiful.

I was so enamored by the Damon System and the beautiful orthodontic cases I saw that day that it was the only treatment I wanted to use in residency. It just so happened that Dr. Damon's son, Paul, was in my class, so we were fortunate to have his father send us twenty orthodontic patients. I will never forget the first set of Damon braces I fitted. After the initial ten weeks of treatment, the patient came back for further treatment. Since my professors had never used this technology, they weren't familiar with the next steps. So I asked Paul what to do next, he called up his dad, and I treated the patient following Dr. Damon's instructions. For the next eighteen months of my residency, that is how I learned to use the Damon System. By the time I graduated in 2000, Damon braces were clearly what I felt would best benefit my patients.

MENTOR, SPEAKER, LEADER, INNOVATOR

Don't wish it was easier; wish you were better. Don't wish for less problems; wish for more skills. Don't wish for less challenge; wish for more wisdom.

~ JIM ROHN

When I completed my orthodontics training and began using the Damon System for my patients, there were really only fifty doctors in the United States using it at the time. Being on the ground floor of the new technology, I took meticulous photographs and records to document what was happening with my cases. Dr. Damon was impressed with my work and my cases, and asked me to share them at Damon forums, starting with the first forum in 2001 and every one since. These days, there are more than a dozen annual Damon forums around the world.

I have now been a presenter and lecturer on the Damon System and the future of orthodontics for almost two decades. For the past thirteen years, I have also been a faculty member at the Redmond Family Orthodontic Clinic at the University of Pacific School of Orthodontics.

I'm also a consultant advisor to medical device companies such as i-CAT, developer of dental and maxillofacial radiography products including an innovative 3-D cone beam x-ray machine (CBCT); Ormco, maker and distributor of the Damon System; Propel Orthodontics, a company that is researching accelerated orthodontics; and Spectrum Lasers, a company that produces lasers for dentistry and other industries. As a consultant to these companies, I work with their engineers and product managers to enhance products by being directly involved in clinical testing. Many of these companies sponsor articles that directly impact the orthodontic profession for good. As an advisor, I document cases with photographs, x-rays, case reports, and PowerPoint presentations to introduce new products and impact orthodontics.

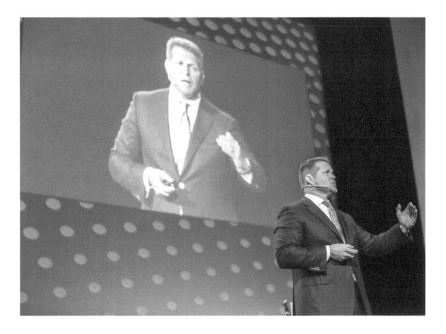

These experiences have given me a front row seat to innovation, technology, and change in the industry around the world. I share these experiences as a lecturer, teaching other orthodontists how to get better at their craft in places as diverse as South America, Mexico, Israel, Germany, Italy, France, Middle Eastern countries, Russia, Dubai, and Australia. In turn, I get to rub shoulders with some of the world's greatest orthodontists, and that has given me a broader perspective on the current state of our great profession.

Meeting so many people and sharing cases has also allowed me to hone my results for patients and, in essence, be a global facilitator: I get to observe other orthodontists and their techniques, employ those techniques in my own practice, improve their efficiency, and share the outcomes of using those refined techniques with other orthodontists to create better finishes for patients worldwide.

It's a role I take very seriously, considering its impact. But there have been challenges. I ask myself, often, why I do this when I have a very busy thriving practice and a large family that needs my attention? Wouldn't my time be better spent here at home instead flying all over the world?

A few years ago, I had been invited to speak in South America and was packing my suitcase when I mentioned to my sixteen-year-old daughter, Meg, that I didn't really want to go. I was exhausted from lecturing around the world while managing a very busy private practice. She looked me square in the eye and said, "You have to go. The people in South America are waiting for you. They need you to teach them, to inspire them how to be better. You have to go." So, I finished packing and I went.

Now, on occasion in these lectures, someone in the audience challenges what I share. The Damon System is an innovation, so it can be difficult to grasp it conceptually—and it can be hard to believe the phenomenal difference in the cases I present. Near the end of that two-day South American lecture, someone in the audience questioned my integrity, stating that I was only there to inflate my own ego. I stopped the lecture. "That's not true," I said and told the audience about the incident with my daughter. "I'm exhausted from all the traveling and running my own practice," I told them, "but I left my home and came here because my daughter told me that you all were waiting for me to help you be better orthodontists. That's why I'm here."

Immediately, people in the crowd stood up and started clapping. I was stunned. It confirmed the commitment that others felt. They felt the passion and the desire I have to help other orthodontists be better.

From that point on, I realized I had a responsibility, almost a higher calling, to teach others and help them be better orthodontists—and I have been blessed to do so.

THERE IS A DIFFERENCE

Be not afraid of greatness. Some are born great, some achieve greatness, and others have greatness thrust upon them.
~ WILLIAM SHAKESPEARE,
TWELFTH NIGHT

When I first began practicing orthodontics, I was, essentially, checking all the boxes by lining up the front teeth and getting a good occlusion (bite). I had no real vision or understanding of what orthodontics could do for people and their self-esteem, but I knew even then that I wanted to be the best orthodontist in the world. I set that lofty goal early on.

Then, about seven years into my practice, my wife loaded our family in the car and we went to have family photos taken, a bit of a frustrating experience as anyone who has ever been through it knows.

However, when we arrived at the studio, I introduced myself to the photographer, who simply replied, "I know who you are." Although I'm from the area, and I know a lot of people in town, I had never met her. So I asked, "How do you know who I am?" Her answer? "You are known as the artist orthodontist."

Her comment stunned me. I'd never heard myself referred to by that name, so I asked her what she meant. She said, "I am the photographer who has been taking photographs of all your patients.

… In fact, I take photographs of many families in the community, and I can tell if they've been your patients because there's a difference in their smiles."

Up to that point in my career, I had never considered myself an artist. I'm not good at drawing or painting. In fact, my handwriting can be pretty hard to read. But hearing that phrase changed my career—`it changed me. Just as Shakespeare said in *Twelfth Night*, I feel greatness was thrust upon me. I now plan my treatments differently. I picture in my mind what I want the final artistic smile to look like. Much as how an artist envisions what the final paint strokes will reveal, I put braces on with the end result in mind.

After that, I started looking at all of my cases as works of art. Instead of just lining up teeth and bringing the bite together, I view every patient who comes to my practice as an opportunity to create a work of art. Through my patients, I have seen time and again how creating a beautiful smile not only enhances facial features but also transforms the whole person.

I wrote this book to help readers understand there is more to orthodontics than straight teeth. And there is a difference in a Frostsmile compared to treatment by other orthodontic providers. I take into consideration what the face looks like and how the teeth relate to the upper lip and smile. Then I design an artistic smile that reflects the light in a way that causes the eye to follow the uninterrupted flow of perfectly aligned and angled teeth from the front of the mouth to the back. A Frostsmile is an eye-catching, almost mesmerizing smile; it makes a person seeing it want to look just a little longer.

Christina, my wife, can attest to that. While we were dating, she asked me a funny question: she wanted to know what made me so special that I taught other orthodontists. "All the orthodontists I know do the same thing: line up teeth," she said. I convinced her to come to a Damon forum in Scottsdale (a few miles from my practice) but didn't tell her that I was one of the keynote speakers. She showed up and sat in the back of the roomful of fifteen hundred attendees, not really knowing what to expect. The lights dimmed, and a song by the band AC/DC started playing over the speakers— "Back in Black" boomed loudly as I started walking from the back of the room with a spotlight following me up to the stage to speak. There was so much energy and excitement in the room that I felt I was floating up to the stage. I delivered an amazing keynote address on creating beautiful faces and smiles using the Damon System. After I finished and came off the stage, I could see Christina standing off to the side while I greeted doctors, answered questions, and even took photos with some of the crowd.

When the crowd died down, she walked up to me, hugged me, and said, "What are you? Some kind of rock star? I get it now." We both laughed. At that time, she was in braces that had been put on by a different orthodontist in our town. Before we were married, the braces were removed, and she opted to let me put her in the Damon System and give her all the finishing touches that have come to define a Frostsmile. That's when she found out what was so special. Now she can see the difference between straight teeth and a beautiful Frostsmile.

Today more than ever, busy mothers are carpooling kids to club sports, they're involved with church groups, and they're seeing all those activities posted online. When they finally get a chance to focus on their children's teeth and focus on their own facial aesthetics and aging, they need to know there is a difference among orthodontic treatments. They need to learn that the care they are getting for their family members and themselves will enhance their facial features and smiles for a lifetime of beautiful aging.

This book is intended to be an insightful guide to next-level smiles. I want you to see how today's orthodontics can help deliver a beautiful smile with far less pain, fewer extractions, in far less time, and with lasting results. It sounds like magic, but it's not. You deserve to know there is a better way than you may remember, and you deserve to know why.

With this book, I hope to inform you with the most cutting-edge orthodontic information based on real-world expertise. As the artist orthodontist for my patients as well as patients around the world, I am dedicated to the endless pursuit of an incredibly beautiful smile for a lifetime.

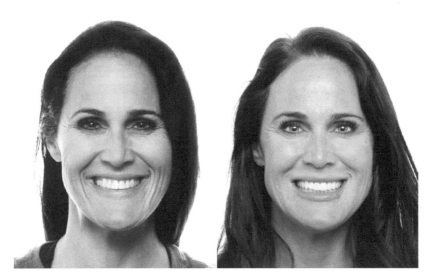

BEFORE   AFTER

CHAPTER 1

A Beautiful Smile: More Than Just Straight Teeth

*The smile is the hallmark
of a beautiful face.*
~ STUART L. FROST

Although my first few years as an orthodontist were all about lining the front six teeth up and getting a good bite for each patient, I later learned that there is so much more to what I now call a Frostsmile.

One of my favorite cases—one that really made me see that difference—was a patient named Ondalynn. When I removed the braces that created her Frostsmile, I saw a different person. Her smile turned out beautifully, but I also realized that something had changed deep inside her. The day I took her braces off, she had a quiet confidence about herself and carried herself differently, almost as if she were a phoenix rising from the ashes.

When she came in for a check-up a while later, I noticed her appearance was different, not just her hair and makeup, but also the way she presented herself. She looked me in the eyes and spoke clearly, with a level of confidence I had not heard in her before. The change in her demeanor made me realize that creating a beautiful smile can be a life-changing experience. More than just straight teeth, a beautiful smile can improve self-confidence and bring joy, happiness, hope, and acceptance. Perhaps most of all, a Frostsmile is empowering. I had empowered Ondalynn to be her best self, a different person from the one she was when she came in for her first consult. That new smile, that new person she became allowed her to connect with other people on a deeper level, something others interpreted as a gesture of love, friendship, and peace.

Ondalynn's transformation was something she had wanted for some time. Although she would have benefitted from braces during her teen years, limited finances prevented her from getting them. I hear this all the time from adult patients who come to see me to transform their smiles. When they were young, their parents couldn't afford braces for them. But now, as adults, they can pay for braces themselves.

Ondalynn was in her mid-twenties before she was able to undergo treatment, and that was when she first came in for a consultation. When I entered the consultation room, I introduced myself and started our conversation by asking her, "Why have you come to see us today?"

She replied, "I'd just like to straighten my teeth."

Unfortunately, she spoke so quietly that I genuinely had trouble hearing her. I almost had to ask her to repeat herself. It was also tough to get her to smile and look me in the eyes on that first visit. In short, the condition of her smile really affected her level of confidence and self-esteem. Here she was, a young woman going to college, working a job, and getting involved in church activities, but her smile kept her from being as open as she might otherwise have been.

As we do with all patients, we took photos of Ondalynn's face, both front and profile views, x-rays using a CBCT, and a full set of intraoral photos, or photos of her mouth. We also took "goop-free" impressions of her mouth to create models (I'll talk more about what it means to be "goop-free" in chapter 6). As with most of our initial exams, our treatment coordinator discussed with Ondalynn her goals for her smile, and talked with her about the technologies we have to offer to help her achieve her goals. The coordinator also talked with Ondalynn about ways we could accomplish her treatments without extracting teeth and without complicated mechanics.

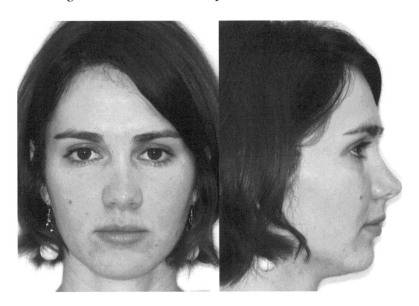

Most patients genuinely don't understand that having braces doesn't just impact their smile but can also enhance their entire face. I explain this during my evaluation, when I look at more than a patient's teeth. Yes, I look at how aligned the teeth are, and the torque (inclination) of the teeth. But I also look at the occlusion (bite), the width of the smile, the arc of the smile, and how much the incisors (front teeth) are displayed in a smile. In addition, I look at how much vermilion (the red part of the lips) shows and how much fullness the lips have. And I look at how the smile relates to the overall facial features.

When I evaluated Ondalynn's facial features I noticed that she had a flat midface with very little vermilion showing.

She also lacked a sufficient border between the wet and dry areas of her upper lip. While a visual exam of Ondalynn's teeth and mouth showed she clearly had multiple issues, it also revealed just how much of a deep bite and a moderate overbite she had and how much crowding there was in her front teeth. Each tooth seemed to be positioned in a different direction.

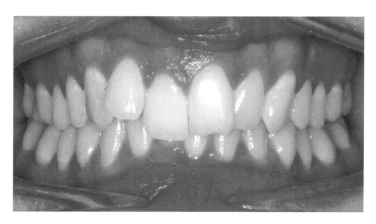

Finally, she had a lot negative or dark space in her buccal corridor, that area between her back teeth and the sides of her smile. The buccal corridor has been found to be a determining factor in what people view as a beautiful smile—less buccal corridor equals a more attractive smile.[1]

---

1   Moore Theodore et al., "Buccal Corridors and Smile Esthetics," *American Journal of Orthodontics and Dentofacial Orthopedics*, vol. 127 (2005): 208–213.

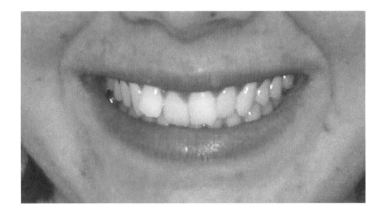

In short, Ondalynn's case was a difficult one, but I was up to the challenge. I'll discuss her treatment and outcomes at the end of this chapter. For now, let's look at one of the reasons people are pursuing a more attractive smile these days.

See Ondalynn's and other
patient transformations at
frostortho.com/frost-smiles

A SELFIE WORLD

We live in a world where people are motivated to look their best, in large part because of social media. People are constantly being photographed these days, and those photos are ending up online for all the world to see. While many of those photos are selfies or shots of people who willingly pose for the picture, it's nearly impossible to avoid having your picture taken at any point in time. Even people who avoid taking selfies are not immune: most people have a smartphone they use to record their every move. Those activities are getting people tagged online, whether they want to be there or not. And with all those photos, people are starting to see features in themselves that they want to change.

So, whether consciously or subconsciously, people are placing more importance on how they look.

In fact, a 2017 survey by the American Academy of Facial Plastic and Reconstructive Surgery found that 42 percent of facial plastic surgeons are seeing patients who want to look better in social media postings.[2]

Many people wanting to look their best start by transforming their smile. They know the value of a beautiful smile as one of the first things people see. One study even found that a great smile is a key feature people equate with happiness, success, and trust. The study involved reactions to images of men and women, and participants didn't realize they were comparing images of straight versus crooked teeth. The results of the study were pretty interesting:

- Twenty-nine percent of the participants said the teeth were what they noticed first.

- Twenty-four percent said that teeth were what they remembered most after meeting someone for the first time.

- Forty-five percent thought a candidate with straight teeth would be more likely to get the job than someone with crooked teeth.

- Fifty-eight percent viewed people with straight teeth as likely to be more successful and wealthier.

---

2   "Social Media Continues to Influence Facial Plastic Surgery Requests," American Association of Facial Plastic and Reconstructive Surgery, news release, June 16, 2017, accessed January 10, 2018, https://www.aafprs.org/media/press-release/20170616.html.

- Seventy-three percent said they were more likely to trust a person with a nice smile than someone who was well-dressed.[3]

Another study published in *USA Today* even found that the male and female participants, alike, rated teeth and the smile as a top priority when looking for a potential date.[4]

Yes, there's a generation of millennials driving social media, but it's spilling over to parents and even grandparents. When older generations see themselves in selfies, or in online posts of a family event, they start thinking of doing something about their smile. Sometimes it's not a photo that drives them but a grandchild making an innocent comment, as kids will do: "Grandma, you've got a crooked tooth," or "Grandpa, you've got a crooked mouth." All of a sudden, they're embarrassed by a smile they've worn for years. And now that they're in a better place, financially, they're ready to get some corrective orthodontics done.

Unfortunately, when people want to better their smile, they sometimes turn to do-it-yourself options. Some 13 percent of orthodontists are seeing an uptick in patients who have tried straightening

---

3   "First Impressions Are Everything: New Study Confirms People with Straight Teeth Are Perceived as More Successful, Smarter and Having More Dates," April 19, 2012, accessed March 7, 2018, https://www.prnewswire.com/news-releases/first-impressions-are-everything-new-study-confirms-people-with-straight-teeth-are-perceived-as-more-successful-smarter-and-having-more-dates-148073735.html.

4   Sharon Jayson, "What Singles Want: Survey Looks at Attraction, Turnoffs," *USAToday*, February 5, 2013, accessed January 11, 2018, https://www.usatoday.com/story/news/nation/2013/02/04/singles-dating-attraction-facebook/1878265.

their teeth on their own.[5] But that can lead to some disastrous results. I hope, from the information I'll share in the pages ahead, you'll see there is a better way.

Since realizing the power of social media, at my practice, Frost Orthodontics, we've started using it to help people see there are differences in orthodontic treatments. I discovered how much people want to know more about orthodontics while I was surfing social media one day. I clicked on an Instagram account that was filled with selfies of women who were showing their braces and talking about their journeys. From there, I started finding a lot of before-, during-, and after-treatment postings across social media. It was interesting to see so many people making what were essentially mini click-through movies that showed the movement and changes in their teeth.

That really hammered home for me how much people are paying attention to what their teeth look like. And it's not just youngsters sharing photos of their braces. It's people of all ages, from young adults in their twenties to baby boomers in their mid-fifties and beyond. People are turning to social media not only to see what other people's smiles look like but also to look for outcomes and results they have not seen before. They're looking at results online and realizing that there are more possibilities than there were in the past. Thanks to social media, people are becoming savvier about what makes for a beautiful smile—and the difference in a Frostsmile.

Today, we post cases online to help spread the word about a Frostsmile. People around the world are starting to see what can be accomplished with today's orthodontics: smiles today are stunningly

---

5   "Orthodontists Report Uptick in Number of Patients Attempting DIY Teeth Straightening," American Association of Orthodontists, news release, February 23, 2017, accessed January 10, 2018, https://www.aaoinfo.org/1/press-room/orthodontists-report-uptick-in-number-of-patients-attempting-diy-teeth-straightening.

different from those in the past. We've had people fly in for treatment from other states, and even other countries, after seeing results posted on social media.

Check us out at
instagram.com/frostsmiles and
instagram.com/drstuartfrost.

A FROSTSMILE— THERE IS A DIFFERENCE

It's unwise to pay too much, but it's worse to pay too little. When you pay too much, you lose a little money, that's all. When you pay too little, you sometimes lose everything, because the thing you bought was incapable of doing the thing it was bought to do.
~ JOHN RUSKIN

What is a Frostsmile? It's far more than just lining up the front six teeth. That's what most people see as a nice smile. But people generally don't understand the difference between lining up the teeth and having a beautiful, spectacular smile.

People often celebrate online the day they get their braces removed: they excitedly post before-and-after pictures on social media. What they don't realize is that, sometimes, the photos look nearly the same. That's because many orthodontists still extract four teeth, line up those that are left, and call it good. They're not really looking at the overall appearance of the smile, how it relates to the patient's face, and how to balance everything.

A Frostsmile has signature characteristics and people looking online for that spectacular finish can see the difference. A Frostsmile doesn't draw attention to any one area of the smile. Nothing interrupts the flow when the eye first sees the front two teeth and then moves toward the back of the smile. Nothing protrudes or stands out from the other teeth because of an odd shape, inclination, or color. When the front teeth are in the correct position, they reflect the light just right to show off the beautiful enamel. The front four teeth hang slightly lower than the cuspids (eye teeth) and when the wearers smile, 100 percent of their upper incisors (front teeth), show while only a minimal amount of gum tissue shows.[6]

And all teeth are properly inclined and aligned. The front teeth don't flare and none are more forward than others—so no "rabbit teeth." From the cuspids to the molars (the teeth on the sides and back of the smile), the teeth are upright: they don't flare out or tilt in. They fill the dark corners (buccal corridor) on both sides of the smile and create a wider, more youthful smile. The jagged edges of the teeth are shaped and the gum tissue is contoured as the final finishes to a stunning Frostsmile.

---

6   Richard Eastham, "Treatment Planning for Facial Balance," *Clinical Impressions* 16, no. 1 (2006): 10–11.

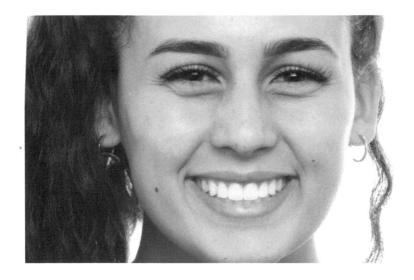

A great smile includes how it relates to the facial features. When the teeth are positioned and shaped optimally, they help create a fuller midface with better lip projection. The midface includes the facial components from the corners of the upper lip to the base of the nose, an area known as Cupid's bow.

Cupid's bow includes the wet/dry border of the upper lip that I mentioned earlier. The wet or red part of the upper lip is known as the vermilion display. A key to a Frostsmile is the curl of that area of the smile. When there's just the right amount of curl upward, more of the vermilion displays. For some people, that makes the upper lip appear plumper from the front, and from the side, it curls upward slightly, making for a very pretty, more youthful look. And when there is better dental substructure, the face ages more gracefully. I'll talk more about how a Frostsmile helps enhance an aging face in chapter 3.

TWO OPTIONS FOR BETTER RESULTS

One of the primary attractions of wearing braces today is that treatment time is significantly reduced. For adults, there are two options. Option 1 is what we like to call a bracelift (as opposed to a facelift). This option is a straightforward treatment lasting twelve to fourteen, or fewer, months to simply align the teeth and broaden the smile to enhance the upper lip and midface area.

Option 2 lasts eighteen to twenty-four months. Similarly to Option 1, this option uses braces to enhance the upper lip and midface. But it also goes the extra distance to correct major issues such as jaw alignment, a gummy smile, a large overbite, or missing teeth. In some cases, this option may include procedures and treatments by other providers, such as an oral surgeon. However, today, there better auxiliary treatments available for children and adults that can help avoid surgery or other drastic measures. For instance, fixing a gummy smile used to require jaw surgery, but today, temporary anchor devices (TADs) can do the job for many patients. Similarly, the braces themselves work differently: they move the teeth with less pressure, allowing for better control over the treatment.

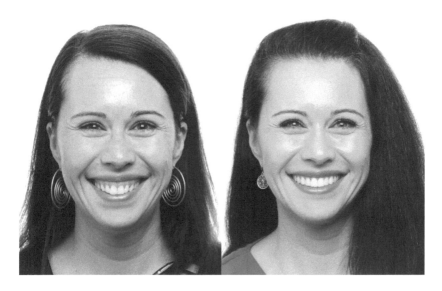

BEFORE   AFTER

With the technologies available today, a beautiful smile is about more than just lining up the front six teeth and closing gaps or eliminating crowding. A beautiful smile really has to do with not just the teeth but also how the smile relates to the face.

THE ART IN A SMILE

*The only thing worse than being blind is
having perfect eyesight and no vision.*
~ HELEN KELLER

Vision and imagination are part of the artist's armamentarium. Just as a sculptor often sees the final work of art before tackling a block of marble, a beautiful smile begins with a vision of how the final result will appear.

Before I put a bracket on a tooth, I envision where that tooth needs to move to create a beautiful, balanced face. By starting with a mental picture of that artistic end result, and then carefully planning the movement of teeth and other facial structures during treatment, we can create a work of art for every patient who comes through the door.

Again, a beautiful smile is about more than just lining up teeth and closing gaps or eliminating crowding. Having a beautiful smile really has to do with how that smile relates to the face as a whole. It includes the occlusion (how the teeth come together when they bite). It includes how much of the teeth and gums show, and how well aligned and positioned the teeth are so that, from front to back, each tooth introduces the next. It includes the shape, condition, and color of the teeth and their relation to each other. And it also includes the arc and shape of the lips in relation to the teeth, and how much of the vermilion shows during a smile. Furthermore, it includes the substructure: the bones of the face that support the smile. That's what helps keep a smile beautiful for a lifetime.

ONDALYNN'S TRANSFORMATION

With that in mind, let me share with you how Ondalynn's masterpiece was transformed from a block of marble to a work of art.

When she came in, she had a class 2 deep bite, which means she had an overbite (the upper front teeth extend too far forward and overlap the lower front teeth). Ondalynn's front teeth completely overlapped her bottom teeth; her lower teeth weren't visible at all. She also had what's known as a collapsed occlusion (bite), meaning that all her teeth were tilted inward.

Using Damon braces, we moved Ondalynn's teeth to where the upper six teeth, from cuspid to cuspid, followed the lower lip line and created a really pleasing smile. Her upper front teeth now hang down over her lower cuspids just slightly, resulting in a really beautiful smile that doesn't draw attention to one side or to one tooth. Her front teeth also have the correct inclination to reflect the light back to the eye of anyone looking at her smile. That creates a smile that inspires people to smile back.

We were also able to straighten up all of her teeth from front to back, from the cuspids to the molars. Nothing flared out, and nothing tilted inward when treatment was complete. That's the hallmark of a Frostsmile using the Damon System: the upper and lower teeth are made broader to allow room to straighten up the teeth instead of leaving them tilted in. As a result, the teeth fill the corners of the mouth (that dark buccal corridor I mentioned earlier).

The Damon System also enhanced Ondalynn's midface, giving

her a nice, upper-lip roll. She shows more vermilion, or more red lip area, so her lips look plumper.

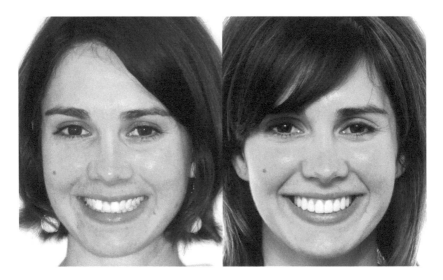

BEFORE   AFTER

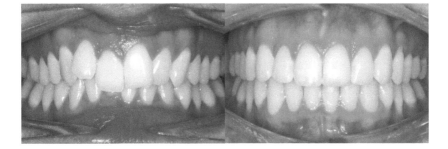

Adults, today, often have what's known as mutilated dentition, or worn, ground-down teeth. Ondalynn started out with a worn notch in one tooth, very pointed cuspids, and one side tooth that really stuck out. With enamel contouring, the teeth edges and chips were reshaped, which added to the youthfulness of her smile.

Once the braces were off, we addressed Ondalynn's gum line, or her gingival architecture. We look at that in all our patients to ensure everything is symmetrical. If needed, we contour the gums to ensure the gum height of the cuspids and two front teeth are the same, and that the gum height of the lateral incisors is not as tall as that of the front two teeth. Once Ondalynn's teeth and other structures were lined up, her gum line looked beautiful. We didn't need to do any gum contouring.

After eighteen months of treatment, Ondalynn was transformed. Not only did she have an amazing smile, a Frostsmile, she was no longer a shy introvert who could barely be heard when she spoke. She was excited and happy to talk with people.

In fact, today, Ondalynn is a spokesperson for our office. She graciously allows us to use her photos to tell her story to anyone who is looking for a change. She wants people to know that the creation of a beautiful smile is a far different experience than it was in the past: the braces are more comfortable, the end result is more pleasing, and the overall experience itself is much improved.

"Had I known about the Frostsmile sooner, I wouldn't have waited so long to transform my smile!"

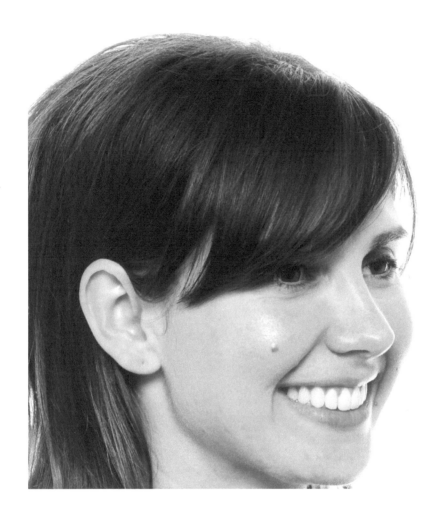

Ondalynn shares her story at
vimeo.com/111473304.

CHAPTER 2

Orthodontics Today: Kinder, Gentler, No More Ugly Metal Braces

*We should not let our fears hold us
back from pursuing our hopes.*
~ JOHN F. KENNEDY

O ften, when we're treating children, the parents will ask questions that let me know they had a less-than-pleasant experience with braces when they were young. "You mean we don't need headgear anymore?" and "I don't want my son or daughter to have teeth pulled" are two of the most common questions I get from parents when I'm treating their child.

If you haven't seen what's new in orthodontics, get ready for a pleasant surprise. Thanks to newer technologies, orthodontic treatment today is kinder, gentler, and more efficient than the treatments of two or three decades ago. No more "train tracks," no more painful bands around the teeth, no more monthly visits, fewer painful extractions, and no more head gear. And, for many patients, no more expander appliances.

Seventeen-year-old Jennifer T. is one example of how a parent's experience made a challenging case even more so.

When she and her dad came for a consultation, he announced, right away, their desire to avoid extractions. "We don't want to pull any teeth as part of her treatment," he said. We often get that same request from parents who had teeth pulled for their treatment a few decades earlier, or who have read online about the pitfalls of extracting teeth. In fact, a number of adults have commented that they had four teeth pulled and now their tongue doesn't fit in the roof of their mouth.

The problem was that Jennifer had some of the most severe crowding I had seen in an orthodontic case in quite some time. There was so much crowding that her permanent cuspid teeth had erupted at almost 90-degree angles from the front of her gums. They looked like fangs, which was unattractive and uncomfortable for Jennifer. The rest of her teeth were tipped in, rotated, and flared; she had multiple issues.

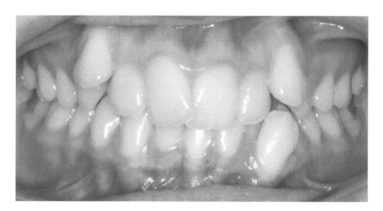

After taking and reviewing the photos of her face (smiling and at rest) and her facial profile, and taking intraoral photos of her teeth, I confirmed how much crowding she had. When I began talking to her, I could also tell that her speech was affected because her tongue was not reaching her palate as it should during speech. She also had a flat midface and therefore didn't have much lip support. This is the area known as Cupid's bow, which I discussed in the last chapter. So even if removing teeth was an option to make enough room to alleviate the crowding, her front teeth would be moved back during treatment, which would further flatten her midface and, over time would negatively impact her facial aging. Yet the goal of treatment is to enhance the facial structures so the face ages more gracefully.

So, initially, there was a little concern about how to treat Jennifer. I knew right away what was needed, but extractions weren't an option. Ultimately, what Jennifer wanted was, in her words, treatment that was "uncomplicated."

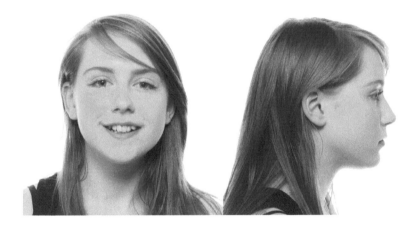

ORTHODONTICS—THEN AND NOW

Orthodontics is a relatively new profession. Orthodontists didn't really start moving teeth until the late 1800s.

Dr. Edward Angle, considered the father of orthodontics, started the first orthodontic college and was all about trying to keep all of the teeth as he was moving them. His philosophy was to widen the smile and avoid extractions.

Over time, the sentiment in the profession changed. Instead of having full smiles and retaining all the teeth, the common belief was to extract four permanent teeth so the rest of the teeth could be moved and treatment would go faster. Back in the 1930s and 1940s, orthodontists believed there would be more stability after teeth were moved if they took out permanent teeth. For another forty years, teeth were removed to eliminate crowding and to stabilize the other teeth. That procedure, it was believed, would eliminate the return of crowding.

Back then, nobody really considered the impact of pulling teeth on the facial profile. But today, we're seeing that patients who have had teeth removed have flatter profiles. In some cases, the extractions even caused some people to have a concave profile: their upper midface is so flat that their lower lip extends further than their upper lip.

Today, the profession is swinging the pendulum back toward treatment protocols that don't involve extractions.

However, many orthodontists are still using the old braces technology, which uses bands to tie the wire to the brackets. In addition to being more painful than modern wires, that act of tying of the wire in place causes more friction and binding during treatment, which ultimately limits the width of the smile. So, to make room for all the teeth, many treatments still involve extracting some teeth.

Many orthodontists also use an expander appliance, which widens the upper palate to make more room for all the teeth. This procedure is possible in very young children, when the suture in the upper palate has not yet fused. (The suture is a seam in the cranial bone in the roof of the mouth. Around age twelve or thirteen, the suture fuses, so expansion is no longer possible.)

Creating a Frostsmile often starts with the Damon System.

The Damon System involves bonding brackets to the teeth and using wire to move the teeth, just as traditional braces do. However, the Damon System brackets are unique. Instead of requiring wire ties or colored elastic ties to hold the wire in place, Damon brackets have "doors" that shut over the wire to hold it in place while allowing it to move inside the bracket. The system is what's known as passive self-ligation (PSL), which reduces the friction and binding between the bracket and the wire, allowing more efficient tooth movement and lighter wires to be used to move teeth. Patient love this new technology because they don't have the pain and severe soreness caused by traditional braces.

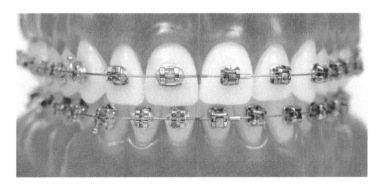

Without colored bands, Damon braces are also easier to clean and maintain, reducing the potential for cavities and white spots that sometimes occur with traditional braces.

The wire itself is also an innovation. It is a high-tech, lighter memory wire that moves the teeth when and where needed.

With the Damon System, there's no need to use an expander appliance to get arch width. Instead, the system itself increases the width of the palate by broadening the arch. In most cases, crowding can be eliminated without having to pull teeth. In fact, in all the years I've used the system, I can count on two hands the number of times I've extracted teeth.

Dr. Dwight Damon, who practiced for many years in Spokane, Washington, invented the Damon System because, after twenty-five years of extracting teeth and treating with tie brackets, he decided there had to be a better way. Although he was moving teeth at a relatively fast pace, that older technology sometimes caused complications with gum recession and bone issues. That's when he came up with the idea of putting a door on the bracket.

His first attempt involved making small metal tubes the size of a braces bracket, bonding the tubes to the teeth, and then threading a light wire through the tubes. He felt that mechanism would more efficiently move the teeth. He tried them on an attorney friend, and six weeks later, was astonished by how much tooth movement had occurred because there was no binding and friction between the wire and bracket. That gave him the idea of creating a tube bracket that allowed the wire to move freely in the bracket slot. The concept involved putting a door over the wire. Instead of tying the wire in place, the door shut over the bracket. That allowed Dr. Damon to change orthodontics forever.

Since there was reduced friction and force, and the memory wire was lighter, tooth movement became more efficient. The treatment widened the arches more, creating broader, more beautiful smiles. And the extra room allowed for far fewer extractions. The system has changed the way the profession is using braces.

In 2000, when I started using the Damon System, there were only about fifty orthodontists worldwide using it. Now there are close to ten thousand doctors using it. Worldwide, only some 35 to 40 percent of orthodontists use some kind of self-ligation bracket.

NOT THE BRACES YOU HAD WHEN YOU WERE A KID

We often hear from adults about how painful their past experience with braces was. Many report that they had pain for days after an adjustment. For some, the pain was so intense they couldn't touch their teeth together to bite down.

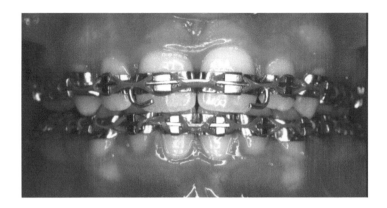

With the Damon System, since there's no tying and binding, there's less pain and discomfort.

That was great news to Eric M. who, at age forty-six, finally decided to get orthodontic treatment for the second time in his life. We had already treated two of his children with great results, so he decided to have something done about the spacing he had developed between his front teeth and we were going to also treat a few other issues.

He had put off having work done, in part because his experience as a teen had been so painful and uncomfortable. But when he saw how beautiful his children's teeth were after treatment, he decided to come in for a consult. It's not uncommon for us to treat parents after they see the beautiful results of their child's treatment.

Eric's treatment was pretty straightforward: We used the Damon System to widen his smile and close the space he had developed between his front teeth. But what was interesting was a comment he made when he came back for the first appointment after the braces were put on: "Wow, these braces don't hurt like the braces I had when I was a teen," he said. "They're more comfortable on my lips, and they're so much easier because I don't have to put bands on them."

In short, Damon braces are kinder and gentler than the traditional braces of two decades ago.

Since developing his original brackets, Dr. Damon has added several generations of brackets, including Damon2, MX, Q, Q2 and D3D. These options allow for more versatile, faster treatment requiring fewer appointments. Another option, Damon Clear, is a nonstaining porcelain bracket that many adults prefer.

Damon Clear was the choice for Jordan L., a fitness trainer who works with people all day long. Working with Jordan was a great fit because my team and I are improving peoples' smiles and Jordan is improving their fitness.

Jordan was hesitant to get his teeth straightened, in part because he didn't want to walk around at age thirty-three wearing "train tracks" on his teeth. But the Damon Clear brackets are barely noticeable on the teeth. In fact, after he posted his experience on social media, a number of people commented that they didn't even know he had worn braces.

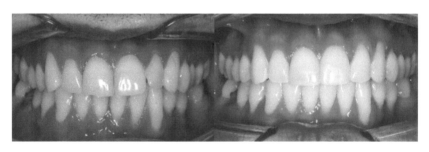

BEFORE   AFTER

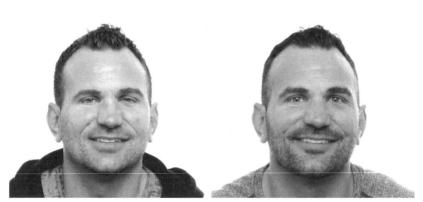

JORDAN LEWIS'S POSTING— DECEMBER 3, 2017

"I was so nervous to get braces at the age of thirty-three. I always wished I had straight teeth but I thought it was too late for me. When I went to see Dr. Frost, I decided beforehand that I probably wasn't going to do it—but everything changed when I walked through the door. When I walked in, they had huge, nice TVs with these crazy, nice massage chairs for the guests to enjoy in the waiting room. Before I even got up to the front desk, the very energetic lady at the front desk said, "Jordan?"

After they took care of me, I got to meet the fantastic and equally happy assistants in the waiting room. Then, I go and talk with doctor Stuart Frost. He was one of the coolest, most straight forward, positive guys I have ever met. I already researched him, so I knew he was the best in the business. I was sure he was going the be outrageously expensive, so I totally was playing hard to get. When we finished talking, I met with the sweet lady to go over pricing and I was shocked how afford-able it was. I got the same quote ten years ago from a small-town orthodontist.

Here's the obvious, I was so impressed with this experience that I had to give them love. They totally changed my smile in less than a year! It doesn't matter if it's your kids or you, they make everyone feel like you're VIP. I can honestly say they have the best customer service I have ever experienced. Thank you, Frost Orthodontics!

PROTECTING YOUR INVESTMENT

Just as treatment protocols have evolved, so have the protocols for maintaining a beautiful smile. In the past, patients were told to wear a retainer only for six months to maintain their new smile, and after that, they no longer needed it.

Unfortunately, without some sort of retainer or retention efforts, many patients relapse. Over time, their beautiful smile returns to its former condition—or worse.

A study conducted by the University of Washington looked at relapse in orthodontic cases and found that to maintain finished orthodontic treatment, it must be retained for life; teeth will not stay in position unless retained.[7] That occurs whether or not teeth are extracted because of crowding.

So, today, retention is all about protecting your investment.

At Frost Orthodontics, we retain teeth for life. We use permanent wires bonded behind the front teeth, upper and lower, from cuspid to cuspid. Then we supply patients with a clear retainer that fits over the teeth and the permanent, bonded wires on the back of their teeth. That clear retainer is to be worn nightly.

JENNIFER'S SMILE

With Jennifer, the solution was to use good brackets and mechanics to widen her arches. That, I believed, would eliminate the crowding of her teeth without having to extract any.

Looking for the artistry in her smile—without extracting teeth—I felt confident I could eliminate the crowding by widening her smile

---

7   Robert Little, Richard Riedel, and Jon Artun, "An Evaluation of Changes in Mandibular Anterior Alignment from 10 to 20 Years Postretention," *American Journal of Orthodontics and Dentofacial Orthopedics* 93, no. 5 (1988): 423–428.

and creating a wider arch. I estimated that the treatment would take between eighteen and twenty-four months. I could see the end result in my mind and I needed to explain to her and her father that we would let the artistry of what I was creating unfold, but we would re-evaluate in nine months. If the treatment wasn't progressing nicely, we would decide whether teeth needed to be extracted at that time.

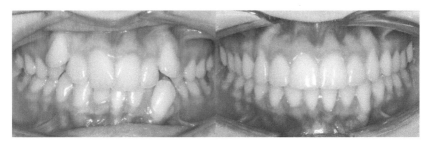

BEFORE   AFTER

Jennifer and her father were relieved, thankful that we were going to do whatever we could without pulling any of her teeth. Since the treatment required visits only every couple of months, it was ideal for Jennifer, who was moving with her father to California and would therefore need to travel back to Arizona for treatment.

In the end, Jennifer's treatment lasted twenty-two months. Damon Q brackets were placed on all of her teeth. When there is severe crowding, as Jennifer had, placing a wire into every bracket can result in teeth flaring forward, which is not artistic. By moving every-thing slowly and tailoring the system to her individual needs, we were able to unravel her crowding and avoid any unwanted movements.

When the braces were removed, her teeth also needed a consider-able amount of shaping and polishing. But since her teeth lined up well and didn't have a lot of surface wear, she didn't need much enamel contouring or any gum tissue contouring.

Jennifer's case really pushed the envelope of what we could do with the Damon System. But, today, she has a gorgeous smile. Her teeth have the right inclinations. Her smile fits her facial features. She has more balance in her face, more midface support, and a shapelier upper lip.

In short, her smile is a beautiful work of art.

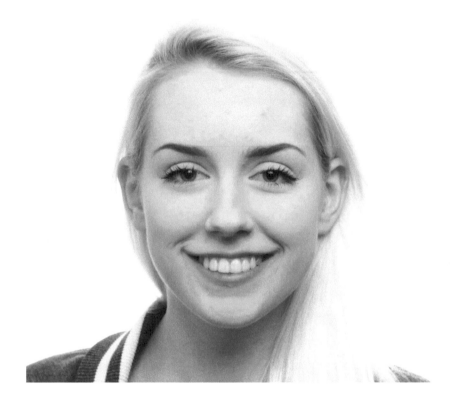

Today, more than ever before, adults who had to forgo treatment as a youngster because of limited family financial resources now have the means to consider a change to their smile. With a Frostsmile, they're getting far more than just straight teeth.

For more patient testimonials, check out
our Smile Gallery at frostortho.com or
go to instagram.com/frostsmiles.

CHAPTER 3

Adult Braces for a More Youthful Smile and Better Facial Aging

If you don't have a smile,
I'll give you one of mine.
~ AUTHOR UNKNOWN

More and more adult patients are coming into my practice with the chief complaint being that they've "lost their smile." They're looking in the mirror or seeing themselves online and realizing that aging is taking its toll and they want to take measures to turn back the clock.

When adults say they've "lost their smile," what they are often describing is multiple challenges. They may have mutilated or worn teeth, a misaligned bite, crowding, problems with their gums, such as inflammation or recession, or even a collapse of the underlying structures of the face due to missing teeth.

Most of the adult patients who present with missing teeth had orthodontic treatment that involved extractions several decades prior.

All too often, the scenario is the same: their teeth are tilted inward leaving insufficient structure to uphold their facial tissue, and over time, gravity has caused their face to age poorly.

The majority of my adult cases need relatively straightforward treatment. For these patients, usually in twelve or fewer months, we can align their bite, broaden their arch to reduce the size of their buccal corridor, and enhance their smile arc. Then there are patients that have multiple issues, some of which can be remedied with surgery, though that is something most don't want to undergo. Today, there are other, nonsurgical options to correct some of the aging aspects that lead to a "lost smile."

Take Mindy S., for instance, whom I mentioned in the introduction. Now let me give you some more details so you can see how her situation came about.

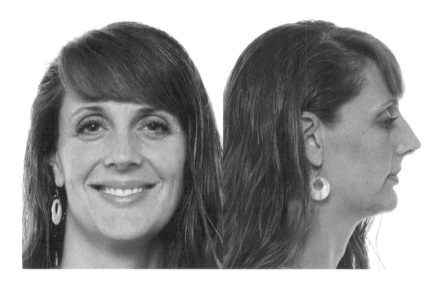

Mindy was in her late forties when she came in for a consult to get back her lost smile. She had already worn braces as a teen. Back then, the orthodontist had pulled upper and lower bicuspids on each side of her mouth to eliminate crowding and then had used braces to move her front teeth toward the back of her mouth. That treatment ultimately created narrow arches and reduced the amount of dental substructure she had to support her face. Over time, she ended up with teeth that were tilted in all around, which had contributed to a sunken-in profile. The problems were even more apparent when she smiled; that's when her large buccal corridor (those dark spaces at the back of her smile) showed. She had so much gum showing in the back that her teeth were barely visible. Her narrow arch was also causing her face to age in ways that were less than attractive.

Many women look to orthodontics to correct aging facial features brought on by the lack of facial support, as Mindy did. They look in the mirror and see those marionette lines on their upper lip indicating that lack of underlying structure. They often find that their lower front teeth have developed crowding and begun to flare out over the years. That happens because of the collapse of the posterior arch. Imagine squeezing the back end of an inflated balloon between your hands. The front of the balloon will push out as a result of the force applied to the back. In the mouth, that kind of squeezing on the posterior arch (the back of the jaw) causes the teeth to flare out or crowd in the front.

The older technique for fixing a large overbite (the upper front teeth extend out and overlap the bottom front teeth) is to extract four teeth, sometimes the upper and lower bicuspids (the teeth on the side of the mouth), and then pull everything in the front of the mouth toward the back. That makes the whole circumference of the arch smaller. The result is a narrower smile and less room for the tongue inside the mouth.

In looking at Mindy's profile, it was clear that she had very little upper-jaw support, which had led to a very flat midface. Her upper lip—from her vermilion to the tip of her nose—was short and flat. The angle of that area of the face should be no more than 90 degrees or it makes the nose appear less attractive. Since her four side teeth were pulled and the front teeth were moved back, the angle of her lip to her nose had changed. In fact, she looked like someone who has had every tooth removed and wears dentures.

Her x-rays also revealed bone loss and gum recession. Often, that's the result of the prior orthodontics using heavier forces to move the teeth.

Ideally, to help restore her smile, Mindy would need to undergo jaw surgery to bring her whole upper jaw, and potentially, her lower jaw, forward. She declined that option, as do most adults who consult me. "What can we do other than jaw surgery to positively impact my face and my teeth?" she asked.

THE IMPACT OF THE AGING PROCESS

Orthodontist David Sarvar has spent much of his forty-year career identifying what orthodontic treatment can do to enhance the face. By studying records of patients from their teen years to their senior years, he has identified what the aging process looks like in a face.

Through his studies, Sarvar has found that the upper lip generally lengthens as people age, resulting in less visibility of the upper teeth. His findings are important for orthodontists to know and consider when working on patients. For instance, when creating a beautiful smile for teens, it's important to take into consideration their smile and face as they age. Anticipating the aging process when creating a youthful smile allows the patient to age more gracefully.

Sarvar also found that the aging face loses volume in the midface, and without the underlying support of the dental substructure, gravity causes the face to droop. That's why the dental arch needs to be broader. A smaller arch lacks the ability to support the facial tissue.

That's what causes aging lines around the mouth.

When considering the artistry of a smile, I try to anticipate that aging process with every patient. That means creating a wider, broader smile in which 100 percent of the upper teeth and up to one millimeter of gum tissue show. In teens, especially, that helps their smile stay beautiful as the lower lip lengthens and gets longer with age.

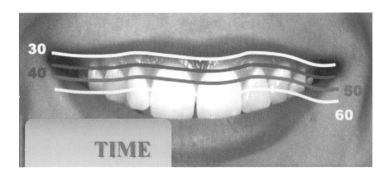

Some adults consider having a facelift to turn back the clock on their aging face. When they come to my practice, they're looking for braces to correct their smile as a way of achieving that goal. But I also use braces and other technologies to enhance their face and help them age more gracefully.

MORE THAN JUST LINING UP TEETH

Adult orthodontics today isn't just about lining up teeth; it's about restoring a youthful appearance—today and tomorrow.

Adults face a number of specific issues with their smile.

Facial tone: As people age and gravity takes hold, the facial tonicity can weaken. Without a strong dental substructure, aging lines can begin to form. With aging, the upper lip also lengthens, leaving less of the upper teeth showing during a smile.

More wear and tear: Adult teeth tend to have more wear than younger teeth. Some adult teeth have unattractive chips and pits that take away from a smile. Fortunately, these issues can be addressed with hard-tissue contouring techniques that restore the anatomy of individual teeth. Hard-tissue contouring can eliminate the need for expensive cosmetic veneers or bonding.

Misalignments: When teeth are crowded, flared, or misaligned, the ability to chew well can be affected. Misaligned teeth can even cause some people to brux (clench and grind their teeth). By aligning the teeth with braces and ensuring each tooth is in the correct position, we can bring back the functionality and youthfulness of the bite.

Gum recession: Adults also tend to face more problems with gum recession. Recessed gums can leave teeth with an unattractive, triangular shape. You've heard the phrase, "He's looking long in the tooth"? Well, that's because the gums have receded and the teeth look longer and unsightly.

Gum recession happens for a number of reasons. Using a toothbrush with coarse bristles can cause gum problems to develop (a soft brush is best for gum health). Regular cleanings at the dentist are also important because food can get trapped below the gum tissue and develop into tartar. Over time, tartar turns into calculus, which acts like acid on steroids to cause inflammation of the gums. That can eventually irritate the bone and cause it to shrink away, a condition known as gingivitis. Gum tissue can only live where there is bone to support it, so when bone is lost, so goes the tissue.

Gingival recession can also occur if the bite is off because the teeth are not aligned. The tooth trauma caused by malocclusion (a misaligned bite), can ultimately lead to bone and tissue loss.

Gum tissue can be recontoured as part of the last steps in a treatment plan. Recontouring the teeth can eliminate the little dark triangle that appears in between the teeth when the gum tissue recedes. Recontouring the teeth and gums fills in that dark space to produce a more youthful appearance.

Narrow arch: When adults have narrowing of the arches due to extractions earlier in life or other causes, the Damon System can return a youthful appearance by widening the arch shape to broaden the smile. A wider arch also allows more room to eliminate crowding or flaring of front teeth. The Damon System is also ideal for straightening up the posterior teeth (the teeth at the back of the mouth), allowing more of the facial part of the tooth enamel to show at the back of the smile. Reducing the amount of gum that shows and the size of the dark buccal corridor creates a more youthful smile.

Less midface support: A broader arch creates a wider smile that balances the face better and creates better upper-lip support. A broader arch also tends to create a better upper-lip curl, essentially plumping the upper lip to allow for more of the vermillion (red part of the lip), to display.

Since a narrow arch can make the face look hollower, a broader smile also promotes better contouring of the cheek bones, which can take years off someone's appearance.

ELLIE'S HOLLYWOOD SMILE

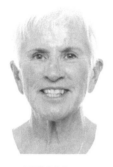
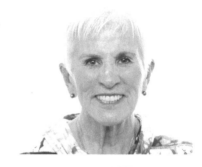

BEFORE   AFTER

Ellie K., a seventy-two-year-old patient of mine, is a stunning example of how a broader, wider smile gives the face a more youthful look.

Ellie's husband was already a friend of mine, and he had received porcelain veneers from a different practice. He suggested veneers to his wife, but Ellie didn't want veneers. Instead, she would "be in for braces," her husband told me year after year. Insisting she was "too old," Ellie put off treatment for some time. But as I tell many patients, "You're never too old for braces."

Still, Ellie didn't come in for treatment until she saw the results of braces on her daughter and two grandsons, whom I treated. And even then, she only wanted "a few teeth straightened." "I don't need a Hollywood smile," she said. Of course, treatment meant aligning every-thing—not just straightening a few teeth—so she opted for Damon Clear braces.

In only a year, we widened her smile and corrected her posterior collapse (the tilting in of her back teeth) and helped her to have a better bite to stop the gum tissue and bone recession that she was experiencing. We also recontoured her teeth and gums to remove dark triangles at her gum line.

Her treatment took five to ten years off her age, and gave her a wider, beautiful smile—a Hollywood-worthy smile.

But even more heartwarming was the text that her husband sent me later: "She just lights up the room when she smiles now."

"I WILL NOT DO BRACES"

Many of the adults who come in for treatment want something to improve their smile without making them look and feel as they did when they wore braces as a teenager. They want braces that don't earn them the nickname of "Metal Mouth" or "Brace Face." Some of these patients are good candidates for Invisalign.

Invisalign is a system of clear plastic aligner trays that fit over the teeth. The aligners are nearly invisible when worn and, as braces do, they work by moving teeth into place over time. Unlike braces, however, the aligners are removed for eating or cleaning the teeth. They are not appropriate for every case, but for patients such as Lesley, for whom comfort was a real issue, they are ideal.

Lesley came in after falling in the shower and incurring a traumatic injury to her front teeth. Her injuries were pretty severe: when she showed up at my office for the consultation, she had already had root canals on the damaged teeth, but her lower lip was still swollen and the remnants of her blackened eyes were still visible. She had fallen forward, which had pushed her front teeth backward to the point that her bite was only connecting on one front tooth.

Biting down on that one front tooth was painful, to say the least, so the last thing she wanted to do was undergo extensive orthodontics. "I will not do braces," she told me in the consultation.

So, we turned to Invisalign, and I created a small retainer to open up her bite until her Invisalign trays were ready. She wore that retainer on her lower arch for a couple of weeks and then began treatment with the aligners.

With Invisalign, we were able to realign her front tooth and even widen her smile. During treatment, we also reshaped her front teeth to remove the dark triangles at the gum line, especially on her lower teeth. When treatment was complete, the damage to her mouth was corrected along with a few other issues, giving Lesley a beautiful, youthful smile.

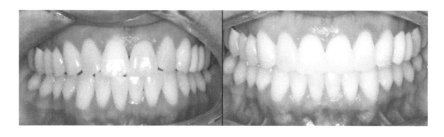

BEFORE   AFTER

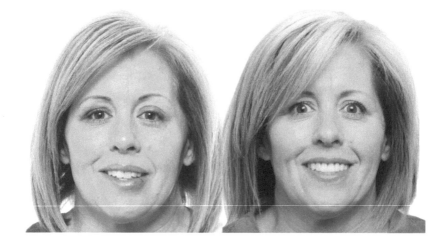

BETTER RETREATMENT OPTIONS

These days, many adults who come in for treatment are looking for faster options with fewer appointments. One study even found that adults are more likely to get braces if the treatment lasts for fewer than twelve months.

When appropriate, accelerated treatments are available that deliver precise, virtually invisible results that can be done in as little as three months.

Accelerated treatments of the past were like hitting a nail with a hammer. Heavy wires were used to move the teeth, and every few weeks the patient had an appointment to get a larger wire applied. The teeth were, essentially, being pounded with a bigger hammer. Not only was that more painful, but that pounding and use of heavy wires and forces may have contributed to some of the destruction seen in some of today's adult mouths.

Today's braces use lighter wires with less friction and binding in the bracket. Adjustments are only needed every couple of months, resulting in fewer visits during the overall course of treatment. And yet the treatment itself is gentler. Again, today's technologies use far less force to move teeth.

Also, the braces aren't as obtrusive. Today's ceramic brackets are far better at resisting stains, making them more discreet, practically invisible (remember Jordan from chapter 2?).

So faster treatment times, less pain, and more comfortable and aesthetic options are reducing the barrier adults face in getting orthodontic treatment.

MINDY'S REVEAL

Now let me tell you more about Mindy's results.

Without surgery, I explained to her, we could use braces to broaden her smile. That, I told her, would enhance her smile but not necessarily to the degree that it would make a significant difference in her facial aging.

Although the other option available to her would take longer, it would open up the spaces where her teeth had been extracted earlier to potentially allow for implants to be placed. That option would, ideally, move her front six teeth forward again to try to reestablish that forward position of her upper front teeth before her cuspids were pulled. It's a very time-consuming procedure, taking as long as twenty-four to thirty months. And it's very difficult because the movements of the teeth must be more closely monitored.

In fact, adult treatments don't always go according to plan. For instance, trying to move teeth to open up space for implants to replace missing teeth might only achieve three-fourths of the space needed. If that were to happen in Mindy's case, as I explained to her, we could put in TADs, which are used along with braces to help move teeth with greater efficiency and more comfort. TADs are today's version of headgear, but instead of being unsightly devices worn outside the mouth and surrounding the head, they are very small devices strategically attached to the jaw inside the mouth.

She opted to move forward with treatment using the Damon Clear system combined with TADs. We moved her upper front teeth forward, carefully watching for any torque or turning of the teeth as we went. We also broadened her arch, which diminished her buccal corridors.

Moving her teeth forward reopened the sites where her teeth had been extracted earlier. Then TADs were anchored behind her cuspids and nickel-titanium springs were used to move her back teeth forward.

After about fifteen months into the treatment, we had opened all the space we could, so it was time to consider next steps. Since it was going to cost about $4,000 per tooth to place four implants in the now-open spaces, she opted, instead, to close the spaces by bringing her back teeth forward using the TADs system.

Mindy's treatment ended up taking about twenty-six months. In the end, opening up the spaces for her missing teeth and then closing the space by moving the back teeth brought the wider part of her smile forward, filling the corners of her smile with teeth. We also straightened up her teeth, which gave her a prettier smile in the back because less of her posterior gums showed. The treatment also improved her bite and gave her more midface support, leaving her with a fuller, prettier upper lip at rest. Her Frostsmile was absolutely beautiful.

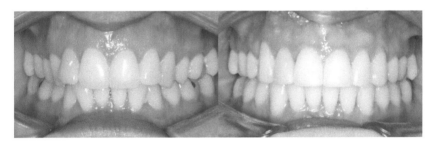

BEFORE   AFTER

When her treatment was complete, I removed all the braces and other devices and contoured and polished her smile. In these last few steps, I don't let patients watch the procedure. Instead, we do "a reveal": I wait until everything is complete before letting patients see their results.

When everything was complete, I handed Mindy a mirror, and I'll forever treasure her reaction: As soon as she held the mirror to her face, she began to cry. She touched her lips and her face and then, with a bright, beautiful smile, she said, "I love it. I have my smile back."

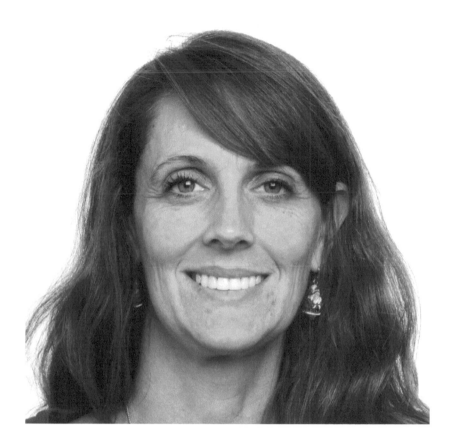

CHAPTER 4

Why Does My Child Need Braces Twice?

An ounce of prevention is worth a pound of cure.
~ BENJAMIN FRANKLIN

What do *phase 1 treatment* and *phase 2 treatment* mean? Does my child really need braces twice? Can't we just put braces on my child once, when all the teeth are in? These are questions I hear daily in my practice from parents looking for treatment for their child. I put this chapter together to help clear up some of the confusion about the two phases of treatment.

For starters, in my perfect world, we would wait to put braces on children when they have lost most, if not all, of the impermanent teeth in their mouth. However, sometimes braces need to be placed on a seven- or eight-year-old to help normalize facial growth patterns and prevent excessive crowding.

Lexi's case is a good example what phase 1 treatment can do for a young child. Lexi was eight years old when her mom brought her in for an evaluation. At the time, Lexi had a bad habit of sucking her thumb. Over time, that habit had caused her to develop an open bite, which is when the front teeth flare out and leave an open gap between the upper and lower teeth when biting down.

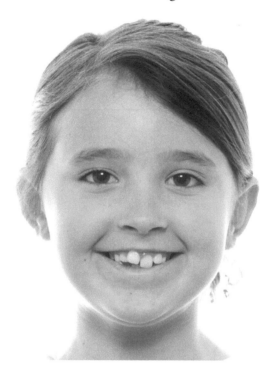

Thumb-sucking habits are very destructive to the teeth and facial structure. During thumb-sucking, the lips create an oral seal around the thumb and the sucking action itself causes enough pressure inside the mouth to force the upper palate or roof of the mouth into a narrow, "V" shape instead of developing nice and wide. All that pressure from the buccal muscles—those muscles on the sides of the mouth—also caused her to develop a crossbite in her back teeth. A crossbite, a form of misalignment, is when the upper and lower teeth don't meet during a bite. In Lexi's case, her lower back teeth were positioned outside her upper teeth when she bit down.

Lexi's high palate also caused other problems for her. When the palate is narrow and V shaped, the tongue cannot reach the roof of the mouth during a swallow. Ideally, during a swallow, the tongue should create a seal that helps push the food and drink down the throat. Since Lexi's upper palate was so narrow, there was no room for her tongue during a swallow. Instead, she would push her tongue forward through the front of her teeth. That action didn't create a seal, so food and drink fell out of her mouth when she ate and drank.

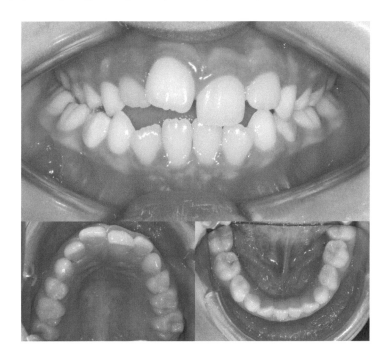

The forward action of the tongue is a condition known as tongue thrust. Since the tongue is a very strong muscle, its constant pushing forward on her front teeth caused them to flare out, creating her open bite. That open bite also caused Lexi to speak with a slight lisp.

During her consultation, she underwent the comprehensive

evaluation using the CBCT and having facial and intraoral photos taken. Then she and her mom sat down with me.

In spite of the problems with her mouth, Lexi had good midface support. When she smiled, nearly 100 percent of her upper front teeth showed, even though they did not overlap her lower front teeth—thus, the open bite. At age eight, Lexi already had her four front incisors, upper and lower, and her first permanent molars were already in place.

Treatment, I explained to her mother, would rebalance Lexi's facial structure and retrain her tongue posture. The age of eight was the ideal time to have Lexi undergo early intervention, or phase 1 treatment.

BRACES—FOR SOME, A TWICE-IN-A-LIFETIME TREATMENT

As I mentioned, parents often ask me why their child needs braces twice. Many children are not born with the ideal orthodontic structure to ensure a good bite and good oral health for a lifetime. While some problems in the mouth can be corrected by wearing braces or undergoing other orthodontic treatments only once, many children need two phases of treatment. Timing is crucial with each of the phases, as is a well-planned, methodical, and customized approach to the treatments used.

One of the best reasons for going through two phases of treatment is that they can shorten overall treatment time. In the past, people wore braces for up to four years. That often caused burnout, leading the wearers to begin neglecting their cleaning and maintenance of the braces. That can lead to the development of cavities or scarring on the teeth due to plaque buildup. By treating twice for shorter periods of time, and with a break in between, the outcomes tend to be far better; they can have a positive impact on a person's health for an entire lifetime.

The American Association of Orthodontics' recommends that all children have an orthodontic check-up by age seven. At that age, it's possible to determine if there are issues related to the child's jaw growth or tooth positions that should be addressed sooner rather than later. Taking advantage of a child's still-developing jaw is one of the best ways to deal with some types of airway issues that are being seen in so many adults these days. I'll talk about this more in the next chapter. Treating a child at an earlier age can help direct orthopedic changes in the jaw while the patient is growing. That's one of the goals of early intervention, or phase 1 treatment.

Interestingly, there is a passionate debate in orthodontics about early intervention treatments in children. Even in orthodontics schools, some instructors are adamantly opposed to any sort of treatment that aligns teeth at an early age. They still adhere to the tradition of extracting baby teeth to make extra room in the jaw for the permanent teeth. On the other side of the debate are those who believe in using the modern treatments available today to make room for more teeth in growing jaws and to move existing teeth into place—often avoiding painful extractions of permanent teeth.

I'm a big advocate of the latter: modern treatments to expand the jaws, retain the teeth, and move them into place or, in the case of baby teeth, slowly extract them as they grow. I believe in evaluating children at age seven and, if needed, having them undergo phase 1 treatment at that time if needed.

Kids who undergo an evaluation but don't need early intervention treatment are monitored every six months at no charge, in my practice, to help determine the right time and options for treatment, and to instill good habits for a healthy, beautiful smile. By evaluating the child at a younger age, treatment can be more conservative and not as invasive. Most of the time, starting young and following up can save time in treatment when all the teeth come in.

Before discussing the two phases, let me share some of the problems that phase 1 and phase 2 treatments address:

Crossbite: a condition in which the upper teeth are positioned inside the lower teeth during a bite. Crossbites can occur in the front teeth (anterior) or in the back teeth (posterior).

Overbite: The upper teeth are positioned outside the lower teeth during a bite. Although a certain amount of overlap is the norm for the front teeth, too much overlap can cause problematic clenching and grinding of the back teeth, which can result in pain in the jaw joint.

Underbite: The lower front teeth overlap and partially cover the upper front teeth during a bite. Underbites may be caused by flared teeth or by a protruding lower jaw. An underbite can affect chewing and speaking, and it may cause jaw joint pain and tooth problems.

Open bite: The upper and lower front teeth are flared forward and do not meet to create a proper bite. Open bite is often caused by thumb sucking or abnormal jaw development. An open bite can cause problems with speech, swallowing, and other functions.

Extreme crowding: Overcrowding occurs when there is not enough room in the jaw for all of the teeth to come in (erupt) normally. Overcrowding can worsen over time, leading to severely crooked teeth, which are not only unattractive but can be difficult to clean. This leads to an accumulation of plaque, which, in turn, can lead to tooth decay and even gum disease.

Impacted permanent teeth: When a tooth is trying to erupt into the mouth in a very crooked position, it can be blocked by another tooth and become impacted. In my practice, we've seen a lot of cuspids, or eye teeth, not lining up in the jaw as they should and therefore becoming impacted.

Underdeveloped or overdeveloped jaws: A patient's facial profile and bite can be affected by malformed jaws and even the airway can be constricted. In fact, one of the primary reasons for phase 1 treatment involves airway and breathing issues.

PHASE 1: SHAPING THE JAWS

In my practice, orthodontic treatment for kids is, generally, fairly conservative. We wait until all the adult teeth have erupted, around age eleven or twelve. At that point, treatment is considered comprehensive, not phase 1 or phase 2. However, when needed, phase 1 treatment can help build a strong foundation for future growth. By correcting the imbalances of the muscles of the face along with any tongue problems or tooth-positioning problems, the structural problems are already addressed, eliminating the need to address them in adulthood.

Phase 1 (early intervention) treatment is crucial for long-term stability of the facial structures. When phase 1 treatment is needed, it can address concerns while a child's bones are developing and growing, potentially avoiding treatment later on in life.

Many seven-year-olds suffer from out-of-balance facial bones and muscles. That imbalance is caused by a narrow upper jaw, jaws too small for the incoming teeth, problems with swallowing or tongue thrust, or other malformations. When we put a very young child in braces or use an expander appliance, we're trying to balance the facial muscles, bones, teeth, and tongue. We're trying to get all those structures to play nicely together.

Phase 1 treatment is carried out when the patient has mixed dentation: a mix of baby teeth and primary teeth, which are the first permanent teeth to erupt. The treatment commonly helps when upper and lower permanent teeth are not coming in correctly or there are other issues associated with jaw size, shape, or position.

The goal of phase 1 treatment is to correct a skeletal problem at an early age while guiding the teeth into the mouth. We want to do everything possible to create, or maintain, space in the jaws to allow the teeth to grow in. Making more room for the permanent teeth to erupt naturally (in a better position) helps to prevent the front teeth from flaring forward or incurring other malformations.

When we address dental issues in children aged seven to nine, we also have the growth factor on our side. In a child of between seven and nine years of age, the palatal suture (the seam in the bone in the roof of the mouth) has not yet fused and become solid bone, so side-to-side expansion of the upper palate is still possible. The child's ability to move that suture can help enlarge the upper jaw and create the space needed for all the teeth to come in. Then, with braces, we can guide the teeth into their proper places.

Enlarging the jaws to make space for all the teeth helps avoid the need for extractions. For instance, if a five-year-old has an underbite, we can take advantage of the fact that the child is still growing and use braces to move the jaw back until it aligns with the top jaw.

Even baby teeth extractions are rarer today. It's more common to place braces on errant baby teeth to slowly guide them into place, and the braces can even help with naturally extracting the baby teeth over time. That kind of treatment allows permanent teeth to erupt in the right position.

Other common reasons for phase 1 treatment these days are airway and breathing issues. Allergens in food and the environment are resulting in more breathing problems in kids, leading to more tooth and jaw crowding and developmental issues. I'll explain how that happens in the next chapter.

Phase 1 Technologies

Early in my practice, I used an older type of braces on phase 1 patients, largely because of cost. When I ran out of the older braces, I decided to put Damon braces on a phase 1 patient. I was astonished at the difference in the arch width after treatment was complete. The patient also had a better-formed facial structure. The outcome was a broader, more beautiful smile with wider arches. Since then, I've used the Damon System on all phase 1 patients.

In the past, phase 1 treatment involved placing brackets and braces only on the four front teeth and on the molars in the back, a treatment known as a two-by-four: two braces in the back by four braces in the front. Today, braces placed on baby teeth helps the arch to develop better, creating more space for the tongue and more room for the permanent teeth. For instance, if a child has a large overbite, we can start bringing the lower jaw forward to correct the jaw position.

The technologies used for phase 1 treatment often include an expander appliance that helps widen the upper palate and promotes better jaw development. Since the roof of the mouth is also the floor of the nose, the expander also helps increase the nasal passages (the airway). Expander appliances are cemented to the roof of the mouth, again, to help open the palatal suture.

Braces in phase 1 are, typically, worn for twelve to fourteen months. Since they involve using lighter wires and movement is slower, with less friction, permanent teeth already in the mouth, or erupting during treatment, remain healthier.

Once phase 1 braces and appliances are removed, the child's jaws are maintained with retainers until all the permanent teeth come in. That's when phase 2 treatment begins.

PHASE 2:
THE ARTISTRY OF THE SMILE

Phase 2 is about shaping the smile and creating that artistic finish. This phase of treatment is the one many people equate with orthodontics: It involves placing braces in a young teen's mouth to line up the teeth and correct any problems causing poor jaw alignment, a bad bite, or gaps and spaces in the teeth. As was the case in phase 1 treatment, one of the goals of phase 2 treatment is to avoid having permanent teeth extracted. So, treatment involves using lighter wires and less force and friction to move teeth where they need to go for the best bite and the most beautiful smile.

In my practice, phase 2 treatment usually begins after all the permanent teeth are in, when the second molars (the twelve-year molars), have erupted in the mouth. Today, most girls at age eleven have all of their permanent teeth; boys have all of them around age eleven or twelve. The treatment usually lasts twelve to fourteen months. In fact, my goal is for most teenagers to be out of braces before they begin high school.

Phase 2 Technologies

The Damon System is used for both phase 1 and phase 2 treatments.

As I mentioned in previous chapters, the Damon System is unlike traditional braces in that it involves closing a door over the areas where the wire sits and allowing for lighter wires and forces to move teeth without having to tighten the braces.

Damon brackets require no ties, so they are easier to clean and maintain. That reduces instances of scarring on the teeth, which sometimes occurs with traditional, banded braces, which are harder to clean.

The Damon System is self-ligating: it uses high-tech, lighter, memory wire to move the teeth with less force and friction, helping the teeth remain healthier throughout treatment.

Since phase 2 also addresses poor jaw alignment, the Damon System is ideal because it widens the upper palate without the need for extractions or an expander appliance.

However, occasionally, phase 2 treatment requires additional orthopedic appliances to help correct some types of jaw malformation, which include:

Herbst Appliance: Patients who have skeletal problems such as an extreme overbite may need a Herbst Appliance to move the lower jaw forward. This repositioning appliance brings the lower jaw forward to balance out the facial features. The appliance is bonded to the back molars, upper and lower, and has telescoping arms that connect the upper and lower jaw. With this treatment, we routinely also place braces on the upper arch to complete the system.

The Herbst Appliance is, essentially, the modern version of the headgear of the past. Headgear, however, was worn mostly at night and compliance was an issue: it only worked if the patient actually wore it. Since the Herbst Appliance is cemented into the mouth, it works twenty-four hours a day, every day of treatment. The appliance is usually worn for around twelve months.

Tongue reminders: Patients who have problems with tongue thrust, swallowing, or a speech impediment (such as a lisp) may need a small, tongue-reminder appliance, bonded in place behind their lower and upper front teeth. This appliance retrains the tongue to rest in the proper position (at the roof of the mouth just behind the front teeth), and to function as is should when eating, drinking, breathing, and sleeping.

A WORD ON COMPLIANCE

When it comes to treating kids, I also think about the parents. The goal of phase 1 and 2 treatment is to take the stress out of the treatment, and to reduce or eliminate the parents' responsibility for the child's care. We don't want parents to have to brush their kids' teeth for them. We don't want parents to have to set timers to remind their kids about a treatment step, as they had to do with headgear and elastics. Our goal is to make the treatment as easy as possible to help avoid burnout of patients and parents as well.

Once the braces and other appliances are removed, the finishing touches are applied to create that signature Frostsmile. In adolescents and teens, that, typically, includes contouring and polishing. If whitening is requested or required, I mostly recommend over-the-counter strips for younger teens. In-office whitening options are available for older teens.

COMPREHENSIVE TREATMENT— FOR ADULTS

Phase 1 and phase 2 treatments for children are different from the treatments we offer adults. If, for example, a thirteen-year-old teen needs orthodontics but has not undergone phase 1 treatment, we consider that child to be a comprehensive treatment patient because all the permanent teeth are in, just as they are in an adult. Many of the adults we treat should have had phase 1 treatment to correct muscle, jaw, or tongue imbalances. They didn't for financial or other reasons. If a child with imbalances does not have phase 1 treatment, those imbalances will still be there when that child becomes an adult, only now those imbalances are causing problems with swallowing, speech, or other functions. Such imbalances are more difficult for adults to overcome than they would have been in childhood at the age of seven or eight.

When structural problems need to be addressed during comprehensive treatment, the same mechanics are used: the Damon System, mandibular repositioning appliances, tongue reminders, or whatever the patient needs.

A GIFT FOR LEXI

Lexi's multiple issues required using braces to widen her upper arch. We also bonded tongue reminders behind her lower front teeth so that when she swallowed incorrectly, her tongue would be uncomfortable and would lift to the roof of her mouth.

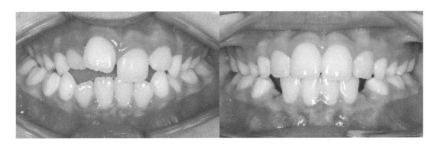

BEFORE   AFTER

Twelve months of treatment broadened Lexi's smile, normalizing her upper and lower arches and eliminating her crossbite. Her bite closes correctly now: her upper teeth properly overlap her bottom teeth. Her swallow has also been normalized and her tongue reaches the roof of her mouth instead of pushing out through her front teeth. She can eat, drink, and swallow—and smile with teeth that meet in the front.

Thanks to phase 1 treatment, Lexi's facial structures can grow normally through all the phases of adolescence. If she had not undergone early intervention, by the time all her permanent teeth had come into place, her mouth would, likely, have had so many problems that proper function would have been hard to recover. She would probably have needed jaw surgery instead of just braces to correct all the damage.

In Lexi's case, treatment at a younger age was medically necessary to improve her swallowing and speech, and to move her teeth into the best positions to promote normal growth patterns. More than that, treatment was a huge gift for Lexi: her facial features and growth are now normalized, preventing her from having serious problems as she develops and grows.

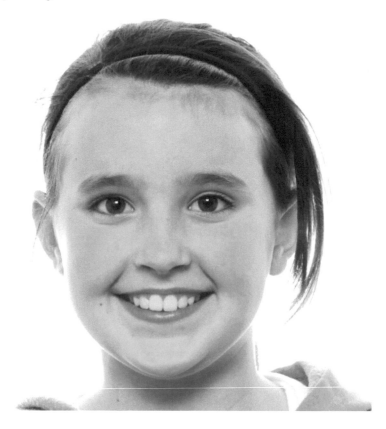

CHAPTER 5

No Child Should Snore: Airway in Ortho

A hero is an ordinary individual who finds the strength to persevere and endure in spite of overwhelming obstacles.
~ CHRISTOPHER REEVE

n July 2017, my family and I were on vacation in Newport Beach. There were nearly two dozen of us there, and at one point, we were all on the beach.

My twin brother, Steve, and I, along with our sons, were playing a game, when my nephew came up to me and said, "This lady needs our help." A woman was standing about fifty yards down the beach, with her hands on her head. She looked very distraught. My nephew told me she had been to the lifeguard station, looking for her missing two-year-old son. Then she had walked along the beach asking people if they had seen her son, but not one person got up to help her.

I told my family we should help her in her search, so we all went down to the where the woman and her son had been together. She was standing on a lip of sand, looking down at the water. We told her we were there to help. "Who are we looking for?" we asked.

"My two-year-old son," she said. "He was wearing a blue swimsuit."

"Where did you see him last?"

"He was right here, digging in the sand."

Immediately, I got a knot in my stomach because I remembered that two years earlier I too was digging in the sand, with my two stepsons, when a lifeguard came over to tell us to fill in our four-foot hole. He explained that someone had died from doing the same thing, the previous month. The hole had collapsed, sucking in the victim, who was buried under the sand.

There were two holes in front of us. I told my nephew to dig in one and I would dig in the other. My nephew pushed two small children out of the way of the hole and began digging.

He hadn't been digging very long when he exposed that blue swimsuit—and the little boy, face down in the sand. I'll never forget the mother's screams as we pulled that two-year-old out of the sand. He was completely gray.

When you're faced with a situation like that, you have to do something. I looked at Steve and said, "We have to begin CPR."

As I held the boy's head in my hands and began removing sand from his mouth, Steve started doing compressions.

As you can imagine, by that point we were surrounded by chaos. The mother was screaming, the father was trying to knock us out of the way to get to the boy to help him, and someone else in the crowd was trying to come forward, yelling, "I'm a nurse. Get them out of the way."

At that point, someone else said, "They're doctors. Leave them alone."

Later, I remember thinking, "Wait, doctors? We're dentists, we're dentists!"

In spite of all that, in that moment, everything seemed to go silent—except my communication with my twin, Steve.

Finally, the little boy's lips moved. "Keep going," I urged Steve. Steve kept giving compressions, and finally, the little boy began to take some tiny breaths.

At that point, the lifeguards arrived and gave the boy oxygen. He started screaming. It was the most incredible, amazing feeling to know that he was going to be okay.

They rushed him away and we were all left standing there, looking at each other as if to say, "What just happened?"

Three days later, we had the opportunity to see the little boy and his family at the beach house we were renting. We got to hold him and take a picture with him. Talk about a glorious reunion.

Just after that incident happened, the story made the news, and the newscasters called us heroes. I've never considered myself a hero. I just acted. But that incident inspired me to be a hero working for my patients.

Especially when it comes to children and breathing, orthodontists have the opportunity to save little children every day!

That's what treatment did for another young patient of mine: Sadie.

At eight years old, Sadie had a lot of trouble sleeping—and it was apparent. When she came in for a consultation, she was lethargic and had trouble keeping her eyes open. She also had dark circles under her eyes, and as she sat with her mother in the consultation, I could see that Sadie was breathing through her mouth.

The photos taken during her evaluation actually told me the story before I met her and her mother: her eyes were half-shut, her mouth was open, and those dark circles were apparent. I had evaluated Sadie's CBCT scan before our meeting and could tell by the 3-D images it produced that she had a severely narrowed airway.

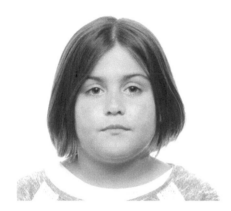 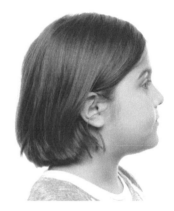

In the consultation room, I wanted to confirm what I had suspected from her photos and test results. As I talked with Sadie and her mother, I saw what I had suspected: Sadie was breathing through her mouth.

I sat down to do a visual examination of Sadie's smile and asked her mother a key question, "Does Sadie snore?" It's a question I ask all parents when I suspect a child's problems are caused by airway obstruction. As is the case with most children,

Sadie immediately spoke up. "No, I don't snore." Since snoring occurs when a person is asleep, it's pretty common for snorers to not even realize they have a problem.

But Sadie's mom contradicted her. "You know what? She does snore," she said. "She breathes really heavy and she breathes through her mouth when she sleeps."

My response? "No child should ever snore."

I kept talking with Sadie and her mom and found out that

snoring wasn't her only problem. Sadie also had trouble getting to the bathroom in the middle of the night, and she frequently wet the bed. But mom had an even bigger concern: Sadie wasn't doing well in school. She had trouble paying attention and, as a result, her grades were starting to fall.

Sadie's snoring, bedwetting, and poor performance in school were likely related to issues that are taking center stage in today's health concerns: breathing problems and sleep apnea.

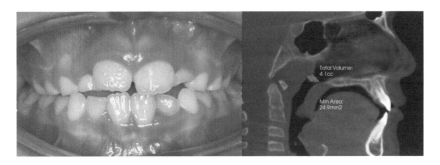

SLEEP APNEA: NOT JUST FOR ADULTS

Sleep apnea occurs when the airway becomes blocked during sleep, causing a pause in breathing. Those pauses in breathing, known as apneic events, often lead to a diagnosis of obstructive sleep apnea.

For adults, there are several options for treating sleep apnea. The most common for severe cases is a continuous positive air pressure (CPAP) machine, which supplies the wearer with a flow of air through a mask worn during sleep. Orthodontists can also create a customized oral appliance to be worn at night. Such an appliance repositions the lower jaw to open the airway and allow the sleep apnea sufferer to breathe.

But children suffering from sleep apnea have another option available to them, one that can permanently change their facial structure to eliminate or reduce the occurrence of sleep apnea for life. I'll discuss this more in the pages ahead, but first, let's look at some of the symptoms of obstructive sleep apnea in children. These are some of the ones we see that help us determine whether to begin our airway protocol to address the issue. Do you recognize any of these in your child?

Snoring: caused by the vibrations of excess tissue blocking the airway. When children snore, we look for a blockage in their airway, from the tip of the nose down to the throat.

Mouth breathing: When there is no room for the tongue to reach the roof of the mouth (the palate), it can rest in the back of the throat and block the airway, or when a child's tonsils and adenoids are enlarged, they can also reduce the size of the airway at the back of the throat. Either of these situations can make it too hard for children to get enough air when breathing through their nose, causing them to open their mouth and jut their lower jaw forward during sleep. In severe cases (like Sadie's), children even breathe through their mouth during the day.

Mouth breathing is a problem because air breathed in should be warmed and filtered through the nasal passages before reaching the lungs. When air flows over the gums and teeth, it dries out the tissues in the mouth, taking away from the natural protection that saliva provides against problem-causing bacteria. Waking with a dry mouth is a problem than needs more than just a drink of water to remedy. It can ultimately lead to inflamed gums and gum disease.

Bruxism (clenching and grinding teeth): If children age seven or eight come in with baby teeth worn from grinding, we know it's because they're not getting enough air. During sleep, and sometimes while awake, their lower jaw is constantly repositioning either side to side or forward to back to open their airway so they can breathe. Again, the roof of the mouth (the palate) is the floor of the nose. When their upper palate is high and narrow, children's nasal passages are affected. But with an expander appliance, we can widen the nasal passages to help a child take in more air when breathing through the nose.

ADD (attention deficit disorder): Sometimes, what is diagnosed in a child as ADD may actually be caused by breathing problems during sleep. Imagine what happens to children who go night after night without getting enough oxygen to their brain during sleep. Eventually, their brain will kick into a state of hyperalertness as it fights to keep the child alive. A child whose brain is hyperalert tends to be bouncing off the walls all the time—at home and at school, or wherever the child goes.

Bedwetting: A brain that is starving for oxygen won't wake a child when the urge to go to the bathroom strikes during sleep. The child will sleep right through any warning signal the brain may put out and wet the bed.

The body needs sleep in order to rejuvenate. Sleep is imperative for good brain function, and good performance in school—and in life. Low levels of oxygen caused by obstructed breathing can, over time, negatively—and even permanently—impact cognitive and brain function and performance. When sleep apnea is not addressed in childhood, it can, over time, lead to health issues in adulthood.

MOUTH BREATHING: A USE-IT-OR-LOSE-IT SITUATION

As I've mentioned, breathing problems are becoming far more common in today's kids—and adults. Allergies to food and the environment are increasing instances of inflammation and even negatively impacting a child's development, reducing the body's ability to breathe normally.

The issue can create a use-it-or-lose-it situation. During sleep, people should breathe in and out through their nose, which filters the air being breathed and also uses the nasomaxillary complex (the upper jaw structures). When children can't breathe through their nose, they end up breathing through their mouth. Breathing through the mouth doesn't use the upper jaw bones and muscles, causing the entire nasomaxillary complex to grow deficient on three planes of space: side to side (the arch width, or width of the smile), front to back (creating an overbite or underbite), and up and down (creating an open bite). Since the roof of the mouth is also the floor of the nose, breathing through the mouth can also lead to the narrowing of the nasal passages, constricting the nasal airway and forcing breath through the mouth. It's a vicious cycle!

When children can't breathe through their nose, they push their lower jaw forward during sleep. That position moves their tongue forward, out of their airway, so they can breathe. Unfortunately, that also means they sleep with their mouth open, creating that whole cascade of issues that comes with mouth breathing.

OPENING THE CHILD'S AIRWAY

The goal of treatment for children with breathing issues is to create the largest airway possible when the child is age seven or eight.

To get a measure of the size of a child's airway, we look at the results produced by the CBCT scan. Those results are recorded in what's known as a minimum constricted area. The number indicates the level of a patient's risk of having sleep apnea. In children, those numbers are:

- 0–50 mm^2 = severe risk
- 50–80 mm^2 = moderate risk
- 80–120 mm^2 = mild risk

When the CBCT scan indicates an airway obstruction in a child, we look at the tonsils and adenoids as potential culprits. Enlarged adenoids or tonsils can block the airway at the back of the throat and make it tough to breathe. That can cause children to push their jaw and tongue forward to open their airway during sleep (back to that whole mouth-breathing issue again).

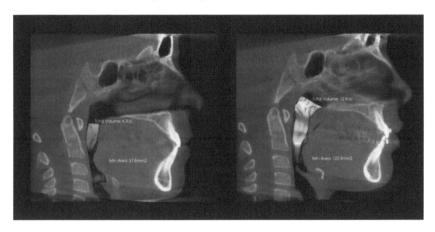

By evaluating the scan results and then getting a good understanding of the symptoms the patient is experiencing, we can create a plan to improve breathing ability by using our airway protocol. For example, if the CBCT scan reveals an MCA below 50, and the patient has symptoms like Sadie's—snoring, bedwetting, and struggling to keep up in school—we may initiate airway protocol by partnering with some outside providers. That may mean sending the scan to a maxillofacial radiologist, a specialist who interprets the imaging and test results and then makes recommendations for treatment. For a child with symptoms like Sadie's, it may mean surgical removal of the tonsils and adenoids and orthodontic treatment with an expander appliance and braces.

As I discussed in the last chapter, the expander appliance opens up the palatal sutures of the face (that seam In the roof of the mouth) to create a bigger airway for the child. Again, we want to take advantage of the fact that the suture has not yet fused, so treatment will involve widening the upper palate or roof of the mouth to also widen the nasal passages.

For many children, expanding the palate triples or quadruples the volume of air they're able to breathe through their nose. In some of the best cases, we've seen a child's airway improve to an MCA of 180 to 200 mm^2 through a treatment plan that included an expander appliance, braces, and surgery to remove the tonsils and adenoids.

Early intervention in airway obstructions is crucial for avoiding sleep apnea further down the road. By expanding a child's palate before the suture fuses, we're able to permanently impact growth phases for the rest of that child's life.

SADIE: A PICTURE OF HEALTH

The treatments we employ for airway obstruction in children are literally transforming their lives—and the lives of everyone around them.

In Sadie's case, we used braces with an expander appliance and, about three months into treatment, she had the surgery to remove her tonsils and adenoids. After the airway protocol treatment was finished, her airway was more than four times what it was when she first came in for a consult.

About a month after Sadie began airway protocol treatment, I received an e-mail from her mother. In the e-mail, she described what it was like to deal with Sadie's issues from a mom's perspective. Her letter was so tender that my wife, Christina, who happened to be in my office when I read the e-mail, cried upon hearing it. She could identify with a mother whose child was suffering but who didn't know where to turn for answers.

Even though Sadie's mother prayed and continually sought medical help for her daughter, she wrote about how inadequate she felt as a mother because her child continued to suffer and was struggling in school. She knew her daughter was smart, even though Sadie repeatedly told her mom, "I'm just not smart like the other kids in class."

Sadie's mother also described how much she dreaded parent-teacher conferences because the teacher kept reporting that Sadie was bright and smart but always looked tired. "She's not applying herself," the teacher would say. "She doesn't seem herself."

Her letter made me realize that what we do in orthodontics goes beyond helping the patient. We're also helping others who are looking for answers to alleviate their loved ones' suffering. Sadie's mother was beating herself up over not knowing how to help her child, not knowing what to do to help her succeed in school. She was so discouraged that she had even considered canceling her appointment with me for Sadie's orthodontic evaluation because she didn't think it would help. Imagine if she had!

The airway protocol (upper palatal expander with upper and lower braces) is a twelve- to fourteen-month treatment. Ultimately, that's all it took to turn Sadie's life around.

Today, Sadie's photos tell a different story. She no longer looks like a tired little girl. The circles under her eyes are gone and she's bright and smiling. All it took was opening her airway so she could breathe and get better-quality sleep. In fact, she no longer snores and hasn't had any accidents during the night. Her life has changed unbelievably.

Even though I have a busy practice and see many patients—children and adults—I try to focus my efforts on making a difference for each patient I see. I believe, and I teach my team, that each of us needs to focus on making a positive difference to the lives of others. We can't change the entire world overnight but should focus on one individual each day. One patient, one team member, or one stranger—that is how we can help others.

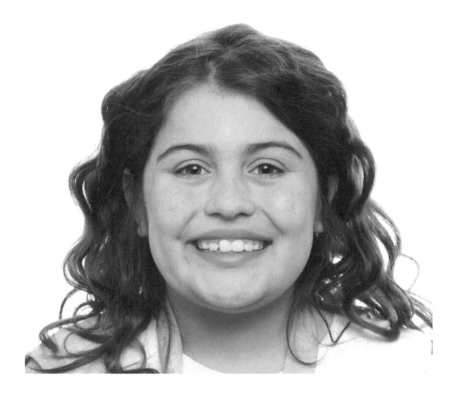

CHAPTER 6

Beautiful Teeth—and Much, Much More

This is not your grandpa's orthodontics! Braces today reach far beyond a band on every tooth and painful experiences.

Forty years ago, orthodontics meant having bands around every tooth and braces with metal brackets that garnered the wearer nicknames such as "Train Tracks" and "Metal Mouth." For some people, it also meant wearing unsightly and uncomfortable headgear. Today, orthodontics has moved way beyond brackets and wires to get straight teeth and a beautiful smile. We have newer technology braces with better wires and other peripherals to produce spectacular results with fewer extractions and less need for surgery to fix major jaw issues.

That was good news for Nicole P., who was so afraid of surgery that she put off getting treatment for many years.

Nicole's journey to fix her smile began about a decade before she came to Frost Orthodontics. She had gone to an orthodontist for a consultation to help fix problems known as gummy smile and severe cant. When she smiled, a good portion of her upper gums were exposed above her teeth, and her smile also showed that her upper jaw and teeth severely tilted to one side. In that earlier consult, she was told that fixing her smile would require more than braces; it would also require surgery to realign her jaw. So she avoided treatment at that time.

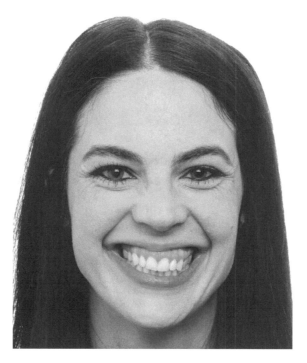

Over the years, she kept looking online to see if any new technology was available to fix her smile without surgery. Then she came across a colleague of mine who offered some of the same treatments that I offer. Since my colleague had moved to another state, he referred Nicole to me.

She e-mailed me about her case, and a few months later, came in for a consult. In spite of having already shared her story with me via e-mail, she was obviously nervous when we first met. She began to relax a bit in the consult as she told me about her situation, and I reviewed her photos and x-rays with her. Since she had been through the standard evaluation at my practice, I had images and a CBCT scan to review with her. That scan showed each individual tooth, the segments of her teeth, her jaw joints, and the relationships between her teeth and facial bones. I also used photos from other cases to show her other patients' finished results to help her better understand how the treatment I was proposing would work for her.

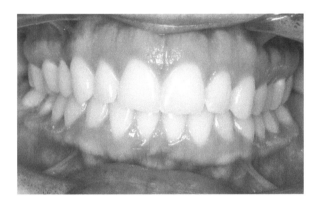

Then I used 3-D imaging technology to show her what I believed we could accomplish, what her finished results could look like. At that point, she actually began crying tears of joy. "I've wanted this for so long," she said, "and it's so exciting to me to finally be able to get something done."

After that, even though she was still apprehensive when I described the treatment, her excitement overcame her fears. In fact, she nervously giggled a few times during the consult at the prospect of getting her smile corrected in under two years.

Her excitement was infectious: I was so excited about the results I knew we could achieve that I couldn't wait to get started. And I was thankful that she trusted me to use my expertise and the orthodontic tools available today to achieve her end results.

ORTHODONTICS: MORE THAN TEETH

Orthodontics goes beyond just lining up teeth. It's about the whole smile: how the upper lip drapes over the teeth, how much gum shows when smiling, how much of the upper lip shows when smiling, and the line of teeth.

Orthodontics also looks at the muscles of the face, head, and neck because they control the way people chew, the way they hold their head—and the way they smile. If these muscles are out of balance, a host of problems can occur. Similarly, if the bite is off, the muscles will fight to correct the bite, which can cause them to become strained. Over time, the excess energy needed to correct a misaligned bite will begin to cause a breakdown of all the affected systems: the bones, teeth, muscles, and so on.

The muscles of the face, head, and neck are also controlled by various nerves. These nerves affect movements of the head and neck along with functions of the face and mouth such as expression and the ability to chew, swallow, and smile. Nerves in the neck also control movement in other areas of the body. That's why dysfunctions in the jaw can sometimes cause pain in other areas of the body.

So orthodontists must understand the anatomy of everything from the neck up and then some. There are dozens of muscles and hundreds of nerves to consider along with the bones and soft tissues of the head and neck. I'm including the formal names of some of these muscles, but what is more important is their function.

Masseter: a large muscle located in the cheek area. It is involved in movements of the lower jaw—specifically, closing the jaw.

Buccinator: a thin muscle located in the wall of the cheek. It is an important muscle involved in smiling, chewing, and speech.

Temporalis: a large, fan-shaped muscle located on the upper side of the head (the temple). It is involved in moving the lower jaw, helping to close the mouth and lips.

Orbicularis oris muscle: a group of muscles surrounding the mouth. They are involved in closing the mouth and puckering the lips.

Zygomaticus major and minor: the zygomaticus major controls a smile, while the minor controls a frown.

Trapezius: a muscle in the back and shoulder that controls arm movement.[8]

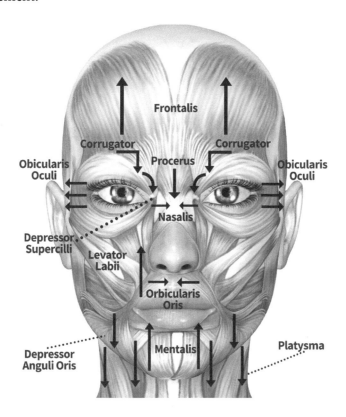

8   "Buccinator," PubMed Health, accessed February 2, 2018, https://www.ncbi.nlm.nih.gov/pubmedhealth/PMHT0030309/.

Why would an orthodontist need to know about a muscle such as the trapezius or shoulder muscle? Because, as I mentioned, the nerves in the neck control other areas of the body. So, if a patient's neck hurts or a patient has a migraine headache, the TMJ (jaw joint) may be the actual cause of the problem, but what the patient is feeling is migrating pain.

Orthodontics is about more than straightening teeth; it also involves understanding how everything above—and sometimes below—the neck works together and creates balance, getting everything to "play friendly" together.

TMJ AND SLEEP APNEA

Since so much of orthodontics is involved in areas associated with the teeth and mouth, diagnosing a problem is a little bit like being an architect of the mouth. It's about understanding how everything works together in order to ensure any "construction" that takes place ultimately makes the entire mouth and face more stable and functional. As with any structure, that starts by ensuring a strong foundation.

The foundation of the mouth is the TMJ, which connects the jaw to the skull. Everyone has two TMJs, one on each end of the jawbone (each side of the face).

Each joint consists of a "capsule," which is where the components of the joint live. It lies where the back end of the jawbone, which is coated in a rubbery cartilage, meets the skull bone. Those bones are separated by a shock-absorbing disc and surrounded by ligaments that support the movements of the joint. When the joint works properly, the disc acts as padding to keep the bones from rubbing together.

When the TMJs are healthy, orthodontic treatment can line up the teeth to provide continued support to help keep the joints aligned over time.

When there's a problem in one or both of the TMJs, the joint can begin to malfunction, leading to a range of symptoms that are sometimes difficult to trace back to the TMJ. Disorders of the TMJ are often caused by arthritis, erosion of the bones or cartilage in the joint, or displacement of the disc by a blow to the head. The symptoms of TMJ can include any or several of the following:

- Pain or tenderness in the jaw joint area, on one or both sides of the face

- Clicking or popping sounds in the jaw joint

- Pain in the head, neck, and/or ears

- Difficulty chewing

- Locking of the joint, making it hard to fully open or close the mouth

- Clenching and grinding during sleep

TMJ problems are often caused by a misaligned bite that can be corrected with orthodontic treatment. By putting the teeth in the correct position with braces and other orthodontic treatments, the muscles can regain balance and reduce or eliminate the extra stress they're undergoing. We're also able to relieve some pain and discomfort with Botox, which I'll discuss later in the chapter.

In addition to TMJ issues, we also come across sleep breathing disorders in some patients.

There are several symptoms that may indicate a patient has sleep apnea (a sleep breathing disorder). In chapter 5 I mentioned those we look for in children: snoring, mouth breathing, clenching and grinding, ADD, and bedwetting. Snoring and clenching/grinding are also symptoms in adults, as are:

- Jerking awake and gasping for air during sleep

- Daytime sleepiness even while driving a car

- Restless leg syndrome

- A neck that is eighteen inches in circumference

- TMJ problems

- Narrow jaw

- Narrow airway

When an adult falls asleep, the muscles of the throat relax and cause a narrowing of the airway, as they do in children. Breathing in may cause the walls of the throat to vibrate, leading to the familiar snoring sound. The narrower the airway, the more vibration and the louder the snore. Adults also clench and grind at night, just as children do, in an attempt to open their airway. That clenching and grinding shows up as wear, broken teeth, and even missing teeth if the problem is severe enough to cause excessive damage.

People who wake up, gasping for air, have a blocked airway; their breathing stopped briefly. The tongue also relaxes during sleep and falls back into the throat to further block the airway and cause those pauses in breathing I mentioned earlier, which are known as apnea.

Narrow jaws can cause sleep breathing disorders because a jaw that is too small to house the tongue can cause the tongue to block the airway. Adults can also suffer from a narrow airway caused by a narrow upper jaw. However, since the palatal suture is fused in adults, expansion therapy doesn't produce the same results of opening the nasal airway. Instead, orthodontic treatment for an airway obstruction may involve a custom-made appliance that is worn during sleep. That appliance moves the jaw forward to help keep the airway open.

With adults, the Frost airway protocol begins with screening to evaluate the symptoms that may indicate a problem or the need for a sleep study. Although orthodontists can treat sleep apnea with appliance therapy, diagnosing it is something only a sleep specialist can actually do—and that is done with a sleep study. The results of the study determine the severity of the sleep apnea, which determines whether orthodontic appliance therapy is a treatment option.

Adults diagnosed with obstructive sleep apnea tend to have other health issues including excess weight, poor diet, fatigue, and even diabetes or heart problems. A lot of that can point back to the fact that they're simply not getting good, restful sleep, because their airway is obstructed.

Recent studies show that obstructive sleep apnea in children is almost as prevalent as it is in adults. Since our airway protocol for children involves expanding the palatal suture, we can usually use our own testing to map out a treatment plan. The larger and more open the airway, the better a person's health will be for the long term. That's why Frost Orthodontics is an airway-aware practice. We want to ensure children have sufficient airways so that as they become adults, they don't fight obstructive sleep apnea and all the health issues that come from repeatedly missing out on a good night's sleep.

ADVANCES TO DIAGNOSE AND TREAT DISORDERS

Today's advances for diagnosis and treatment are making orthodontics more efficient, more comfortable, and a better experience overall. With these new adjuncts, we can better diagnose problems. And if we can diagnose better, we can treat better, leading to the best outcomes. Here are some of the advances that we use at Frost Orthodontics.

Cone beam computed tomography (CBCT): As I've mentioned throughout the book, one of the advances we use to diagnose patients today is a cone beam, technically known as a computed tomography (CBCT). The CBCT is a three-dimensional x-ray that produces very detailed images to help us assess and pinpoint problems of the structures in a person's body from the neck up. The unit rotates around the patient's head and captures data using a cone-shaped x-ray beam. The data collected is then used to reconstruct a 3-D map, of sorts, of the teeth, mouth, jaw, neck, ears, nose, and throat. It's an advanced tool that lets us see far more than older technologies in a fraction of the exposure time. The information we gather from the CBCT can help us create more precise plans for treating the jaw joints, impacted or missing teeth, and airway obstructions from the tip of the nose to the throat.

The CBCT uses about as much radiation as a panoramic dental x-ray, and as much as 95 to 98 percent less radiation than medical CT scanners. Companies such as i-CAT or Imagining Sciences have reduced the amount of radiation from the CBCT to be equal to walking in the sun for a few hours.

3Shape digital scanner: With our digital scanner, we can skip the goopy impressions of the teeth. The digital scanner uses a wand equipped with a video camera to capture images of each tooth and create a detailed, digital map of the teeth, arches, and gums without having to endure a dreaded mouthful of mush. The scan takes less than five minutes. The digital impressions created by the scanner are then threaded together to create a 3-D digital model of the teeth, gums, and bite of both the upper and lower jaws.

Once the digital copy is created, it can be printed out as a 3-D plastic model of the patient's mouth, just like the plaster models that used to be created using the goop as a mold. The model is then used to create Invisalign and other custom appliances that are more precise than those created with the goopy plaster casts of the past, and with a faster turnaround time.

The plastic models are presented to patients at the end of their treatment as part of the Frostsmiles for Life program. If patients break their retainer, the dog eats it, or they toss it away in a napkin at a restaurant, they can bring in their plastic model and we'll use it to create a new retainer, free of charge.

The software also allows for digital manipulation of the teeth to help visualize movement and show how treatment will progress.

Botox: These treatments are offered to patients experiencing headaches as a symptom of TMJ issues. Many of our patients struggle with headaches and migraines because their bite is off and they have some form of TMJ or facial muscle problems. Our goal is to use braces to move teeth into the best position to balance the muscles of the face, which can reduce or alleviate headaches and pain. For patients who continue to struggle with headaches because the TMJ muscle is stressed out, we offer Botox treatments to temporarily shut down some of the muscles that are causing the headaches or TMJ issues.

Botox has become a regular offering in our practice to bless the lives of our adult patients. The treatment lasts for around three months.

Spectrum laser: This device is ideal for contouring the gum tissues following treatment. I start the contouring treatment by using a topical gel to numb the gums, and then I use the laser to ensure symmetry from side to side. I follow a very methodical approach to get the correct proportions of the gum tissue architecture along the upper front teeth: I make sure the central incisors (middle two teeth), are 1 mm higher than the laterals (the teeth on either side of the incisors). Then, I make sure the cuspids (the fangs) are the same height as the middle two teeth.

There is a temporary burning sensation from the treatment. I liken the pain level to burning your mouth when eating hot pizza: the gums may burn for a brief time, but the irritation is easily forgotten in a half hour or so. The treatment itself lasts a lifetime.

The laser is also used to make room for teeth that are erupting in the mouth. For instance, if a cuspid is impacted and causing problems with crowding, and with other teeth trying to come in, the laser is used to remove the gum tissue and uncover that impacted tooth. A bracket is then placed on that tooth to gently guide it into place.

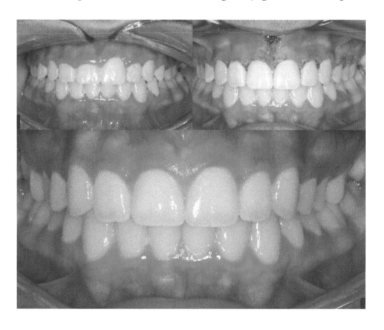

VectorTAS temporary anchor devices (TADs): Only a decade ago, the fix for a problem such as a gummy smile was an invasive jaw procedure by an oral surgeon to move the jaw up. Today jaw surgery is avoidable by using those amazing TADs I mentioned in chapters 1 and 3. TADs are very small devices strategically connected to the braces and anchored into the jaw to move the entire jaw or certain segments of teeth to fix issues such as gummy smile. TADs move teeth with greater efficiency and more comfort. Essentially, they function as did the headgear of the past, but they are placed *inside* the mouth where they are often unseen.

Invisalign: A lot of adult patients are asking for Invisalign, the clear aligner solution to straightening the teeth. Invisalign is a system of clear plastic aligner trays that are changed over time to move the teeth, as braces do. Unlike metal braces, however, the aligners are nearly invisible when worn. Many of my adult patients looking to straighten their teeth wore braces when they were kids or teens. But their treatment relapsed, often because they did not continue to wear their retainers. While they'd like to have their teeth aligned again, they're not willing to go through wearing braces. So, now clear aligners available.

Today, more than ever, we have amazing technology for moving teeth and creating beautiful outcomes. In addition to the Damon System, we have other advances available to help patients avoid jaw surgery, extractions, and long treatment times—all while creating the most beautiful smiles.

NICOLE'S SMILE: THE PERFECT BALANCE

For Nicole, treatment consisted of placing Damon braces on her teeth and working up to a strong, stable arch wire. We also placed TADs on one side of her mouth and attached springs between those and the braces to raise up the teeth that were canted down. That works because, as the teeth move back up into the gums, the bone surrounding the teeth remodels to support them, and the gum tissue rises up with the teeth.

When I sit down with patients, I listen to their chief complaint and overlay that onto what I see is needed to create a Frostsmile for them. In examining the artistry in Nicole's smile, and aided by the data from the CBCT images, I was able to envision the end result before placing her brackets and TADs.

Once the treatment began, I saw Nicole every couple of months to ensure everything was on track, as I do with all my patients. During those visits, the bond between orthodontist and patient tends to strengthen, adding to the trust factor. That turned out to be especially significant with Nicole.

After twenty-one months of treatment, it was time to remove her braces and TADs. Usually, I remove them in one visit and then wait three weeks to contour teeth enamel and gums to get the architecture of the smile just right. But Nicole was so excited to get to the final result that she agreed to be one of my patients at an in-office course that I offer twice yearly for other orthodontists. So, with a dozen orthodontists watching, Nicole let me demonstrate how to remove braces, contour her enamel, and then contour her gums.

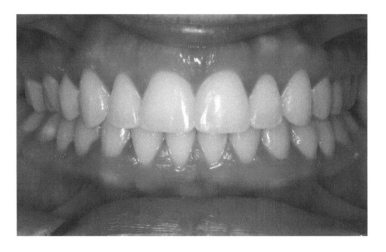

When the procedures were completed, Nicole sat up and smiled for the camera—an amazing Frostsmile—and we recorded it all on video.

The treatment not only leveled the cant in her smile but also widened it. In addition, the treatment leveled her gum tissue and reduced the amount of it that showed. Now, she only shows about one or two millimeters of gum tissue from side to side. The end result is a beautiful, pleasing, balanced smile.

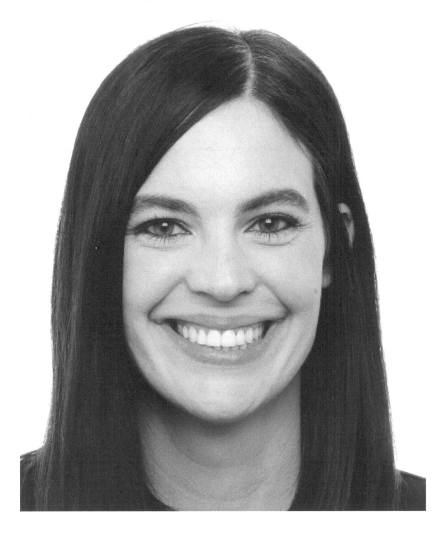

We posted Nicole's before-and-after photos on Instagram and the commentators—including other orthodontists—are just blown away that her results could be accomplished without jaw surgery. Instead of being admitted to a hospital and undergoing a very invasive procedure, everything was done in our office with no more numbing than a touch of gel. We used our office technology to understand Nicole's issues, determine the best course of treatment, ensure accuracy in bracket and TAD placement, and then monitor and guide her progress. All it took was fourteen appointments over twenty-one months to create the balance Nicole had longed for.

By now, I hope you see that what we do is more than just straighten teeth. We really go above and beyond to create something truly spectacular. That's what happened in Nicole's case.

For more patient testimonials, check out our Smile Gallery at frostortho.com or go to instagram.com/frostsmiles.

CHAPTER 7

The Specialty of Orthodontics: There Is a Difference

THE FROSTSMILE

When it comes to orthodontic treatment, there is a difference in turning to a professional who has undergone the training to produce the outcomes a patient needs and wants.

Currently, the American Dental Association states that a general dentist can offer patients treatment in an oral specialty by getting a little extra training. With a weekend course or two, dentists can offer services such as the removal of wisdom teeth, a procedure usually done by an oral surgeon. They can perform a root canal, a procedure usually done by an endodontist. And they can offer to install braces, including brackets or clear aligners such as Invisalign. In fact, today, general dentists can offer treatment for just about anything that other professionals specialize in—professionals who have undergone years of training to learn their specialty.

Oral care specialists such as orthodontists spend two or three years beyond their general dentistry training in full-time academia: schooling and hands-on patient care. That's a minimum of two years just learning the essentials of a specialty. After training, they spend their days providing treatment to patients in their area of specialty.

Now, let me be very clear: I am not against general dentists installing braces. In fact, I've seen some very nice smiles that were created by a general dentist using braces.

But some general dentists have trouble understanding the limits of their role. They struggle to recognize when a patient's needs are beyond the scope of what they learned in a weekend course. As a result, instead of sending complicated cases to a trained and qualified orthodontic specialist, they often attempt to take on such cases themselves—and sometimes with disastrous results. That has begun to strain what was once a good relationship between the general dentist and orthodontist communities.

The situation really began to get complicated during the Great Recession of the mid- to late 2000s. When the economy started to tank, the dental industry as a whole took a real downturn. People began putting off dental work because it was an expense they felt they could forgo for the sake of other needs. During that time, general dentists began adding Invisalign to their treatment offerings to try to keep patients coming in the door.

But the truth is that Invisalign is more complicated than just placing clear aligners on teeth. That's starting to become more apparent now with some patients who have completed the treatment with less-than-optimal results and had to seek out an orthodontist for further corrections.

I myself went back to school to learn orthodontics after

practicing general dentistry for five years. I didn't want to just dabble in orthodontics; I wanted to be taught the proper techniques through proper training. While I was practicing as a general dentist for five years, my twin brother, Steve, was training as an endodontist (a root canal specialist). He had a real talent for doing root canals when we were in dental school together, but he didn't stop there; he went on to get specialized training.

Let me tell you a story of how that makes a difference. After training as an endodontist for two years, Steve came back and set up his own practice in the community where I practiced general dentistry with our father. Shortly thereafter, I had a patient who needed a root canal, so I sent him over to my brother to have that procedure done. It took one visit, one hour, for my brother to perform that root canal on the patient. Afterward, the patient came back to me and thanked me for sending him over, "I am so thankful you sent me to your brother. He was awesome. It went very fast," he told me.

At that time, it sometimes took me two or three times as long to perform a root canal—the same procedure my brother was able to do in one hour's visit. Plus, sending a patient to a specialist for treatment strengthened my relationship with this patient: he returned to me, very happy with his care. I remember thinking back then, *why would I ever do another root canal when someone else can do it better than me? Why would I even try when there is someone else more skilled who can give the patient an excellent experience?* At that point, I decided all my root canals would go to my twin brother, who was a specialist and could perform them better than I could, while giving my patients exceptional care.

Again, to be clear: I have great respect for general dentists; they have to be skilled at dealing with many different types of oral problems. And I am not against general dentists installing braces. I have seen some good outcomes from braces put in by a dentist.

But then there are cases such as Amanda B's.

When Amanda came to Frost Orthodontics for a consult, she was wearing braces with clear brackets. She had already been in treatment for eighteen months but came to see me because she didn't really like the way her smile looked. She could tell something wasn't quite right, even though her general dentist had told her he was removing her braces in two weeks. So, she came to me for a second opinion.

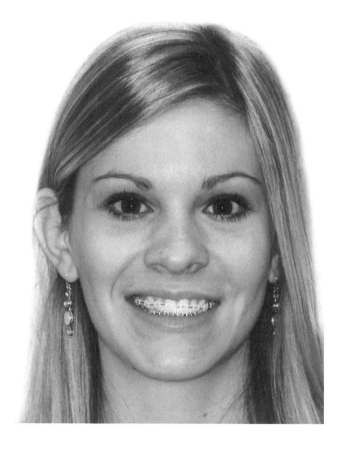

When I reviewed her tests and sat down with her for a consult, she told me she didn't like the fact that some of her teeth didn't fit together. She said her teeth looked as if they were "on different plains of space." In other words, she felt they were not all lining up the way they should in relation to each other.

I looked at her teeth and, sure enough, her upper cuspids were angled in and the front teeth were too upright. In other words, there were some torque problems with her teeth. The wire being used on her teeth was round, which is not the best choice in finishing wire. After eighteen months, Amanda was unhappy with her results, and she had already spent the same amount of money for treatment as she would have spent with me.

THE ORTHODONTIST DIFFERENCE

Amanda's experience is not that uncommon, and it happens because of the differences in training and experience among providers. In Amanda's case, and in many similar cases that I've seen, the provider just doesn't understand some of the subtle techniques that are best handled by a specialist: bracket placement, torque, and facial balance, among others. Plus, Amanda didn't understand that not all providers are specialists. She was led to believe that braces were a specialty, not just a sideline, of the general dentist who had treated her.

Cases like Amanda's are emotionally tough, in part because they remind me of my experience in general dentistry where I sometimes dealt with teeth after a provider had stepped out of his or her realm of expertise. And it breaks my heart to have to tell patients who have already spent thousands of dollars on treatment that they have to spend thousands more on retreatment to get the results they were after in the first place.

That happened to Toni, just before Christmas one year. A general dentist, who was out of his realm, had put Toni in Invisalign for two years but had not achieved her desired results. So, she came to me and we came up with a treatment plan using the Damon System. It took another twelve months of treatment to get her the smile she needed and wanted. She was in treatment for three years, instead of two, and, essentially, she paid for treatment twice.

That kind of case is frustrating for everyone involved.

Look at it from the perspective of traditional medicine. Your primary care physician may recognize when you have a suspicious mole. He or she may even have the tools to remove that mole. But if that mole were on your face, would you want your family care physician to remove it? Or would you rather be referred to a plastic surgeon, someone who specializes in dealing with facial aesthetics, to reduce the chance of ending up with an ugly scar? What if that mole turned out to be cancerous? Would you want your primary care physician or the plastic surgeon to treat you? Or would you rather be referred to an oncologist, someone with specialized training to deal with your disease?

Again, orthodontics is about more than just moving teeth, and moving teeth is about more than just placing a bracket somewhere on a tooth and adding a wire. A beautiful smile comes from years of training and experience, using the latest technologies, creating a customized treatment plan, monitoring the progress of that plan to its completion, and performing those signature, finishing touches. That's what is behind a Frostsmile.

WHAT TO LOOK FOR IN A PROVIDER

Unfortunately, people don't always realize that the provider they have chosen is not an orthodontist but someone offering orthodontics as a sideline. Here are some things to look for in a provider to ensure that he or she is truly someone who can deliver the results you need and want.

Training and experience: Instead of choosing a provider based on training or skill, patients often choose an orthodontist because their office is near their home or because a family member or friend referred them.

Again, an orthodontist is someone who has specialized training beyond dental school. In that two- to three-year period of training, the orthodontist is taught head and neck anatomy, tooth structure and function, the way teeth move, how the bones of the face and teeth relate to each other and work together, and special techniques for treatment. As you can see, there's a lot to learn, more than can be learned in a weekend course. And that training includes hands-on experience in working with patients.

Choosing a provider based on a personal connection can cloud a person's judgment. It can be difficult to question the treatment given by a provider who is also a neighbor or referral from a friend.

A modern practice: Orthodontic treatments today are more advanced than treatments of the past. But unless orthodontists are continually on the lookout for the latest advances, they will get behind on the best treatments for their patients. I like to be on the cutting edge when it comes to technology in orthodontics. If I come across orthodontists getting better results than I'm getting, I want to learn about what they're doing. I may even camp on their doorstep to find out what they're doing and how they're doing it.

A modern practice keeps up on the latest technologies. When combined with expertise, these technologies lead to more accurate diagnoses, faster treatment times, better outcomes, and a more efficient process overall.

The ability to teach others: It's one thing to know your craft and another to be able to show others how it's done. Orthodontists who teach tend to have a better understanding of the skill because they have to explain it, in detail, to others. Plus, teaching is a little like sharpening the saw: it makes the orthodontist hone in more on the details when treating patients, resulting in better outcomes.

I've been teaching for more than a decade in the orthodontics department at the University of the Pacific. I also fly around the world and teach other orthodontists how to be a great orthodontist. Those interactions allow me to also learn from others, which helps me enhance my own skills. I can improve on that new information with my own patients and take that knowledge out into the world to advance the industry as a whole. I always want to improve on what I learn, not because I want to be better than someone else but because I believe the student should eventually be better than the teacher. That's what defines a great teacher.

A plan for protecting a patient's investment: Orthodontic treatment is an investment, one that needs to be protected for a lifetime. An orthodontic practice should have a retainer program to help patients keep their smile for the rest of their lives.

At Frost Orthodontics, we bond permanent wires behind the upper and lower front teeth, and supply patients with a retainer that is worn at night. We also have a "retainers-for-life program" to replace retainers that are lost or destroyed.

Early intervention for children that also addresses the airway: Does the practice offer phase 1 and phase 2 treatment for children? If so, does the evaluation in phase 1 also include an evaluation of the airway? The goal of phase 1 and phase 2 treatment should be more than just aligning teeth; it should look at how treatment will enhance the patient's life for the long term.

When the airway is constricted in a child, a few months of

specialized orthodontic treatment can open the narrow airway, preventing sleep apnea when the child becomes an adult and improving overall health.

An orthodontist is a physician for the mouth. If a child—or adult—can't breathe because of an obstruction in the airway, an orthodontist can identify whether a patient needs further evaluation, treatment through a partner provider, or an oral appliance to correct a structural issue.

Adult orthodontics: Some orthodontists focus primarily on children and don't offer much in the way of treatment for adults, if anything at all. In truth, it's more fun and a little easier to work on kids. They tend to go along with treatment pretty willingly, without questioning much.

Adult treatment can be more difficult, however, because the patients often ask questions. In their eagerness to see change, they may look in the mirror several times a day just to see if anything is different. If one tooth doesn't appear to be moving, they'll question it at their next visit. They really like to know the details of their treatment, so it can take more energy and effort than treating a child. All of that takes more time, and it takes someone who cares enough to truly listen and provide answers.

Adult orthodontics may be more complicated because adult teeth have been exposed to life's wear and tear, movement can be more difficult than in a child's mouth, and adult health is often less than optimal.

But adult orthodontics is more rewarding because it is so transformational. Some adult patients have gone their entire lives with crooked or missing teeth, or other oral issues. And to finally get those addressed is truly life-changing for them. Adults are often more emotional than kids, because they're seeing a dream come true after so long.

Hands-on treatment and finish: Several appointments are made during the treatment process during which the orthodontist's hands-on care is especially crucial.

One is when the brackets are placed and bonded to the teeth. It's critical that brackets be placed in the right position to ensure the best outcomes, and that's something a trained and experienced orthodontist should do—not an assistant.

Another is the midcourse correction. About halfway through the process, the orthodontist should review updated x-rays to check the positions of the brackets to ensure they're correctly placed and to review the roots of the teeth to ensure they are in good health. If adjustments need to be made at that time, again, the orthodontist should move the brackets—not an assistant.

Finally, at the end of treatment, after the braces come off, the orthodontist should apply the finishing touches by contouring the enamel and gum tissue, as needed. By allowing an assistant to do these steps, the orthodontist is missing out on the artistry of a smile, the opportunity to create something really beautiful.

An optimal start: Anyone with a little training can bond brackets to teeth and place wires on the teeth to line them up. But there is a difference when it comes to creating an artistic smile. In orthodontic school, we're taught the intricacies and details of the mechanics involved in moving teeth and creating a balanced face. The goal of any treatment with braces should start with optimal placement of the brackets to have the optimal, balanced smile and facial structure when the braces come off. Bracket placement can reduce the need for additional treatments at the finish, such as gum contouring.

A great finish: Over time, I have developed an eye for what truly looks beautiful at the end of treatment. A lot of that goes back to the five years I spent as a general dentist. I started really noticing the shape of teeth while working with veneers (porcelain teeth that are available in the ideal shape and contour).

That ideal is what I strive for when applying the finishing touches to each tooth at the end of treatment, which can be tricky. While children's teeth often need little in the way of contouring at the end of treatment, adults often have teeth that are worn or misshapen by use. It's my job to return the youthfulness, the ideal shape to each tooth, whether through enamel or gum contouring.

So, a Frostsmile creates that artistry by addressing the ideal in each tooth individually, how each tooth relates to others, and in the smile as a whole. That starts with placing the brackets, and finishes with shaping the front teeth and gums to complement the line of the lips.

When gum contouring is needed at Frost Orthodontics, it comes as part of the treatment itself without additional charge.

Proof of outcomes: When choosing a provider, look for one who is proud to show off results, whether on an in-office wall of fame or, perhaps more importantly, online.

At Frost Orthodontics, we have no shortage of patients who are excited to show the world their Frostsmile. They happily post their results on their own social media sites. And they let us post their before-and-after photos on our sites as well.

> Want to see our outcomes? Check out our Smile Gallery at frostortho.com or go to instagram.com/frostsmiles.

The go-to for other professionals: Is your choice of orthodontist someone other professionals turn to? At Frost Orthodontics, we count among our patients other orthodontists, local general dentists, and the family members of these professionals.

We also have patients from around the world. We've treated people who have come specifically to us from across the United States, Canada, Mexico, and from even as far away as China!

An amazing team: A visit to the orthodontist should be a pleasant experience, one that includes being greeted and cared for by an amazing, talented, and trained team.

The team members at Frost Orthodontics love what they do, and it shows in the patient experience. They're super nice, work well together, make patients feel like family, and have a passion for creating amazing Frostsmiles.

AMANDA'S OUTCOME: A SMILE FOR A LIFETIME

Remember Amanda from the beginning of the chapter? After I explained to her and her mother what they could expect with the end result, they consented to move forward with treatment. I removed the braces she was wearing and placed Damon braces on her teeth. In twelve months' time, she finished with a beautiful Frostsmile, one that she was happy and proud to wear.

Again, the artistry of the smile is about more than just lining up teeth; it's about creating beautiful smiles that transform lives. That's something I take very seriously. My goal is to create something so spectacular that it changes patients on the inside, giving them self-confidence and a smile they can be proud to wear the rest of their life.

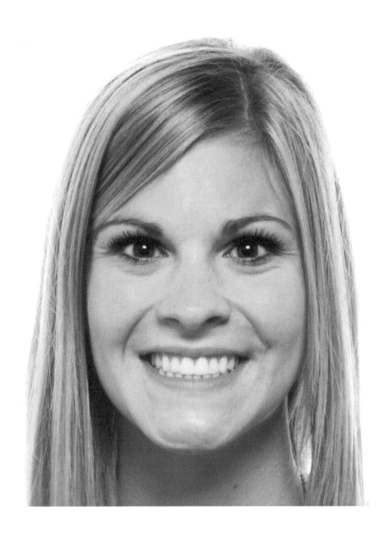

Conclusion

I love it when you smile, but I love it even more when I am the reason behind your smile.

~ AUTHOR STUART L. FROST

J ust as there is a huge difference between braces put on by general dentists and braces put on by orthodontic specialists, there are also many differences in the finished results from one orthodontist to another.

Remember I mentioned in the introduction that Christina, my wife, can now see the difference? She'd had braces fitted by another orthodontist when I met her, and she didn't realize that there is more to a smile than just straight teeth. She thought, at that time, all braces were the same; all produced the same results. But after going through treatment a second time, using the Damon System, and under my guidance, she now sees the difference when she looks in the mirror—and she sees it when she's out in the world.

Now, I didn't set out to be an artist in orthodontics. But I earned that reputation because I care about patients and their results. I start every treatment by first looking at the patients and seeing the artistry of their smile as I'm evaluating them. And then I push the envelope of what I can do to help bless their lives, to really give them the benefit of my training and experience.

Admittedly, there are times when patients don't participate in the treatment: they're not keeping their teeth and braces clean, they're not using their elastics as needed, and they're not exercising good judgment when it comes to the food they eat. Simply put, they're not doing their part to create a beautiful smile.

To ensure the best outcome, it's imperative for every patient to take an active role in treatment. All patients should follow the treatment plan recommendations, watch what they eat and brush and floss regularly. Without those good oral hygiene measures, cavities can form under the braces and scarring white spots can form around the brackets. At the end of treatment, their teeth may be straight, but their smile won't be its best because of those marks. Lack of good oral hygiene can also cause the gums to become irritated if food and plaque buildup on the teeth, leading to gingivitis and extreme swelling that can cover the teeth and disrupt and prolong treatment.

While there is an amazing difference in a Frostsmile, the experience itself is one that places patient comfort at the forefront. That's something I learned from working alongside my father for five years. He had a gift for making all the patients who sat in his chair feel they were the most important person in his life at that moment. Yes, he was known for his love of material things—especially a nice car and watches—but what he valued most were the relationships he made throughout his life. At the end of the day, he knew that was all that really mattered.

For me, it's the same. When I meet patients at their first appointment and they become excited about how the treatment is going to change their life, I get excited too. Then I get to spend another year or two treating them and getting to know them, and they become almost like family. After the braces come off and they see their beautiful Frostsmile, they realize that we've been on a journey together, that we've worked hard and created something they will have for life. I often see patients for ten to fifteen years after treatment, and they still have their beautiful Frostsmile—and the memories of our experience come back again. That's part of the reason I love what I do.

It's also about transforming lives. I remember that when I was a general dentist, I helped a patient who had overlapping front teeth by giving her what she wanted: four beautiful, sparkling veneers on her front teeth. While she was elated, I felt empty inside because I hadn't straightened her teeth and created something beautiful and lasting. That's why I became an orthodontist: I wanted to create lasting changes. It's my greatest desire for people to recognize a Frostsmile, whether on someone else or on their own face when they look in the mirror.

People who come away with a Frostsmile are transformed. They are more self-confident, they smile more, and they really enjoy life— and with good reason: they have a new outlook and a smile that will last them a lifetime. Every time I see patients look in the mirror and see their Frostsmile for the first time, I am reminded of the life-changing gift my father gave to me many years ago. I realize now that he was the one who gave me the very first Frostsmile, which has left a lasting legacy not only to me but to all my patients. Thank you, Dad!

If you, or someone you know, are in need of orthodontics and can see the Frost difference, reach out to us at frostortho.com. Together, we will create a Frostsmile for life!

Our Services

t takes an incredible team to deliver the kind of patient experience people have come to expect at Frost Orthodontics. This is a group of talented professionals with a vision for community, passion, and teamwork. We love what we do, and we work together to create truly beautiful Frostsmiles. We go above and beyond to ensure your treatment experience is as wonderful as your finished smile!

Treatments we offer include:

- Damon System braces
- Invisalign
- Early interceptive treatment
- Adult treatment
- Accelerated treatment
- Advanced technologies including TADS and laser gum contouring
- TMJ treatment, airway and obstructive sleep apnea treatment
- A Frostsmile finish

Reach out today to schedule a consult:

5058 E Southern Ave, Suite 101, Mesa, Arizona 85206
Smiles@FrostOrtho.com 480.325.7500 www.frostortho.com
instagram.com/frostsmiles facebook.com/frostorthodontics